Managing Stress
in Veterinary Medicine

Managing Stress
in Veterinary Medicine

Allison Johanson

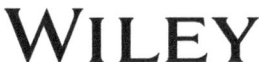

Published by John Wiley & Sons, Inc., Hoboken, New Jersey.

For general information on our other products and services or for technical support, please contact our Customer Care Department within the United States at (800) 762-2974, outside the United States at (317) 572-3993, or fax (317) 572-4002.

Wiley also publishes its books in a variety of electronic formats. Some content that appears in print may not be available in electronic formats. For more information about Wiley products, visit our website at www.wiley.com.

Library of Congress Cataloging-in-Publication Data
Names: Johanson, Allison, 1986– author
Title: Managing stress in veterinary medicine / Allison Johanson.
Description: Hoboken, New Jersey : Wiley, [2026] | Includes index.
Identifiers: LCCN 2026004850 (print) | LCCN 2026004851 (ebook) | ISBN
    9781394331970 paperback | ISBN 9781394331994 adobe pdf | ISBN
    9781394331987 epub
Subjects: LCSH: Veterinarians–Job stress | Stress management | Veterinary
    care teams–Job stress | Burn out (Psychology)–Prevention | Resilience
    (Personality trait)
Classification: LCC SF756.28 .J64 2026 (print) | LCC SF756.28
    (ebook) LC record available at https://lccn.loc.gov/2026004850
LC ebook record available at https://lccn.loc.gov/2026004851

Cover Design and Image: Wiley

Set in 9.5/12pt STIXTwoText by Straive, Pondicherry, India
Printed and bound by CPI Group (UK) Ltd, Croydon, CR0 4YY

C9781394331970_140426

This book is dedicated to all of the people who came before me as healers. For countless generations, the work of healers has informed the work that I do now. I would also like to thank my kids and my husband for dealing with me while I wrote this book.

Contents

Appendix

Foreword

In vet school, there were always meetings with opportunities to talk to professionals throughout the industry. As students, we would show up in droves to glean whatever small bits of information we could to help form a picture of what life might look like after leaving the familiarity of the classrooms and the safety of each other's company. It didn't hurt that almost all of them served free food and we were very broke.

At almost every one of these meetings, the speaker would say, "If you would have told me ten years ago that this is what I'd be doing, I wouldn't have believed you." As someone who went to school to study dairy cows, the Labradors of the large animal world, I remember wondering to myself over and over: *What am I going to be doing 10 years from now?*

Imagine my surprise when, now a little over 10 years out, I find myself a small animal veterinarian who, in addition to clinical practice, works in continuing education and can't remember the last time I put on a pair of coveralls and rubber boots.

It was through my continuing education work at VetFolio where I met Allison. Usually, in the process of creating a piece of content, there is an initial call where the speaker and I get to know each other and formulate a few talking points. All I knew going in was that we were talking about mental health in veterinary medicine.

Mental health has been a large topic of conversation in VetMed over the last several years. To me, it seems to be a conversation that has done a great job identifying the causes of mental health challenges, but not so much when it comes to practical solutions. To be honest, going into this call, I was prepared for an erudite and overly conceptual conversation about "forming boundaries" and "practicing self-care."

My preconceptions were quickly quashed once Allison and I started talking.

I was met with someone who was about as far from snobbery and grandiosity as you can get. She was warm and felt like somebody I'd want to go have a beer with. Despite not being a veterinary professional herself, she had clearly done her homework. She didn't lead with a lecture on the larger problems we're all too familiar with. Instead she was focused on what went on for us day-to-day, minute-to-minute, and I could tell she had spent time helping people who needed to implement real change without overhauling major aspects of their lives. This was someone who was here for the real conversation.

Over the ensuing weeks and months as we made content together, I continuously had to remind myself to focus on the broader audience. Allison made it so comfortable to want to talk about my personal experiences. And I wasn't the only one who felt that way.

I remember doing a webinar with her and watching the comments continue to roll in well past our ending time. People were connecting to her message and trying to glean as much insight as possible, much like those meetings from way back in vet school (unfortunately, webinars don't come with the free food). Allison's approach was so relatable. It wasn't a talk about "getting enough sleep" or "buying a gym membership." It was a much deeper dive into the unique trauma we experience in VetMed, and how to address it in ways that don't require taking large amounts of time off work or focusing on going to bed earlier.

Several months later, after navigating a separation, closing my mobile business, and overhauling my career to shift toward emergency medicine, I've spent a fair bit of time in therapy myself and have reached for many of Allison's techniques to get me through moments of panic and overwhelm. So when she reached out, telling me about this manuscript and asking if I'd write the foreword, the answer was a no-brainer. I am so honored and grateful to play even a small part in supporting her work.

Before I'd finished the preface, I found the same honest, humble, and funny person I had met on that first call. The information is well-researched and the words paint an accurate picture of many of my experiences in VetMed, but the delivery still felt like talking to a friend. Like unloading at the end of the day with someone who really "gets it," but who (bonus points!) also has the training and insight to make the challenges seem more manageable.

The message found in these pages is one of validation and reassurance. It is a reminder for all of us who love this wonderful, terrible, rewarding, and challenging field that while in VetMed the sailing is rarely smooth, we already possess many of the tools we need to navigate the challenges and continue to find joy, longevity, and balance; we may just need someone like Allison to come along and provide the map.

Cassi Fleming, DVM

Preface

While Trauma therapy is a large part of my job, trauma work is not all that I do. I also work with people to resolve personal life struggles. I enjoy working with healthcare professionals as they start feeling burnt-out or notice a disconnection with people they love. Many do not come to my office to work on burnout, but they come due to interpersonal struggles, depression, or anxiety. Through exploration and therapy work, we learn to define it as burnout. People often assume burnout is unrelated to the other symptoms they want to heal. When literature talks about burnout, it frequently describes it as something very obvious when you are going through it. Healthcare systems also convey a message that you are just supposed to live in burnout; it is part of the job. This is especially true in the higher-stress healthcare professions, like veterinary medicine. This message is debilitating. It implies that if you sign up for the passion-driven job you feel called to, you have to be miserable in all parts of your life. No wonder there is cynicism, retention problems, and low well-being scores. This message has to change. We need to establish hope, coping strategies, and a culture of care for each other. We need to meet the expectation of positive well-being and purpose in our careers. Misery is not the only solution to a high-stress job. Yes, you may have to work harder to regulate the go-go-go nature of the job, and you may have to create some intention in caring for your nervous system as it moves from one thing to another, but with practice, that gets easier. Habit takes time, and we are building habits here.

In addition to the "suck it up, it's part of the job" mindset, I have also seen a lot of information about preventing burnout that conveys that if you experience it, it means you are weak. It isn't usually said, but it is strongly implied. Messages that suggest burnout is caused by not exercising enough or not managing your emotions well enough convey this message. If you go to supervisors in specific clinics and express concern about burnout symptoms, you are told to "do more self-care" or "Start prioritizing yourself." These comments are great in theory. Yes, it is essential to exercise and prioritizing yourself is necessary, but burnout is much bigger than this. In the throes of burnout, the simplicity can sound invalidating and create shame. These messages can also downplay the significance of the symptoms and their impact on daily life. I do not believe that anyone is intending to create harm by discussing the struggle in this way. I do not believe these concepts are wrong in any way. I simply think they're missing some significant components of the big picture.

While work-related stress is not "just part of the job," it is likely to come up. You can develop all the skills, maintain good health, and work hard to enjoy your job, yet you may still experience some of the stress responses discussed in this book. Heck, you might even get burnt-out on trying so hard not to burnout. The key is to notice it before it gets too big and have a plan for managing it when it comes up. The knowledge provided in this book can help you navigate burnout without having to leave the job you've worked so hard to get. If you choose to leave, you can do so based on what is best for you, rather than emotions that feel unmanageable. You are not weak because things are hard; you are human and working in a difficult field. You are not weak because you did not know these skills earlier; you cannot know what you don't know. Life gets hard, skills fall short, and all of us are fallible, especially within the context of well-being. You deserve to live a life closest to your best, authentic self, and this book can help.

Spending many years as a trauma therapist and being pretty geeky about the content, I have gained a wealth of knowledge about how the body responds to a traumatic situation. Like any geek or someone who truly loves the nature of their job, I have surrounded myself with advanced learning throughout my career. Due to my interest, much of my advanced training focuses on natural, bodily reactions to stress and trauma. I noticed and learned that when people go through stressful events in their lives, they can present with symptoms similar to those of animals in the wild. People label these reactions as depression, anxiety, feeling stuck, burnout, etc. Our bodies are not very good at telling the difference between real and perceived threats, and respond similarly. If we were out hunting and gathering berries and a saber-tooth tiger presented itself, we would react in a way that would keep us safe. This is how we have survived as a species for all these years. Our body responds similarly to emotional threats as to physical threats. Our nervous system has labeled specific thoughts, emotions, and situations as a saber-tooth tiger. This reaction can be very confusing to the cognitive brain. We know logically that we will not die from a situation, but our body responds in a way that it might.

Sometimes, stress responses are a single incident that disappears and feels insignificant over time. We finish the natural cycle of safety response. Sometimes, the reactions are chronic and seem incapable of determining what is safe. They become stuck in a perpetual lack of safety. These chronic responses create vigilance, and you rarely feel secure, even if you cognitively know you are safe. This response is unconscious and spontaneous. No one is asking it to happen. It just happens. I wonder if the system never found the safety needed to escape this emotion because the threat continued over time. I know that you likely know that you will not immediately die from the stress of your job. Long-term consequences are known to create health concerns, but this safety part of our brain is hypothetically saving us from immediate threats. The messages we learn throughout life teach us that unmet expectations, specific emotions, and mistakes will shun us from the tribe, ultimately killing us. Our brain has not evolved to fit the complicated life we live today.

While these concepts apply to the therapeutic office, of course, I found that they also apply to workplace stress, including burnout, compassion fatigue, and vicarious trauma. I am not discrediting the difficulty of traditional trauma. It can manifest in more complicated, challenging, and intense forms than workplace stress. However, the responses can also be very similar, so similar concepts apply. The body's systems appear to perceive something in the workplace as a threat and respond accordingly. Noticing this connection was a relief, as I can now use the techniques that work so well on trauma on a broader group of people. But why does this happen? I hypothesize that the body responds to the stress because the work is designed to be fast-paced and stressful, with little time for rest in the workplace. This creates hormones in the body that allow for survival in this environment. People never learn how to come down from the rush of the day, and eventually, their bodies become exhausted. The body then learns that the work poses a threat to its system and perceives it as such. Alongside this, individualism gets lost in the hubbub of the workday. People start to feel unseen, lonely, and unimportant. If this doesn't make sense, don't worry. I will go into more detail in the nervous system section of the book.

So why work with veterinarians? At some point in my journey, a veterinarian stumbled into my office. She felt like she needed a drink (or several) after getting home; she felt stuck and unsure of what to do about it. She felt undervalued by the handlers and exhausted from the day-to-day work of a veterinarian. As time went on, she started feeling better, and we decided to discontinue treatment, both moving on. Fast forward, a month or so, and an article popped onto my desk. It spoke about the struggles with mental health and suicide in the veterinary field. Being the person I am, I began to dive into a rabbit hole of research around the battle with well-being in veterinary medicine. I started asking myself why veterinarians are twice as likely to struggle with mental well-being as other healthcare professionals and four times more than the average population (Pohl *et al.,* 2022). Those are big numbers. As I researched and learned, I noticed that my expertise with trauma seemed to be weaving in, and it started to make sense to me. I began teaching CEs and speaking to veterinarians about managing their well-being from my perspective as a trauma therapist and a nervous system geek. From a nervous system perspective, the research makes sense and creates aha moments for those listening. I became passionate about helping veterinarians make sense of their struggles so that they can gain skills to keep them in the field and thriving. My goal is to establish hope for a fulfilling life in veterinary medicine.

When I was asked to write this book, a published book was not on my list of goals in my life. I reviewed my mission statements for myself and my career. One of my priorities as a therapist is to provide creative ways to be assessable. Well-being and mental health are still stigmatized in our society. People still sheepishly come to therapy, hoping no one sees them walk through the door. Many times, people wait until loved ones give an ultimatum or they feel like there is no hope before making changes for their well-being. I hope that this book allows for a foot in the door to change. I hope that people can build resilience to manage the hard parts of their careers and lives. I hope that when people hit a difficult time, they have a place to turn that feels less threatening to gain skills toward change. I hope that this book allows more people to create a life where they are responding and living in the best way possible for them. Most of all, I hope we can start conversations toward saving lives.

Allison Johanson

REFERENCE

Pohl, R., Botscharow, J., Böckelmann, I. and Thielmann, B. (2022). 'Stress and strain among veterinarians: A scoping review', *Irish Veterinary Journal*, 75(1), p. 15 https://doi.org/10.1186/s13620-022-00220-x.

Acknowledgements

To all of the veterinary professionals I have had contact with throughout the years. You are truly a hidden paragon. Praise is minimal, actions are unseen and misunderstood, and yet you continue on carrying out your work to the best of your ability. You are an inspiration to all helping professionals.

To all the researchers and professionals who came before me, paving the way for the knowledge I can provide in this book.

To my family, who encouraged me throughout the year of the book-writing process. They never protested or questioned when I had to take time out to write. The pride and encouragement are endless. I feel grateful to be able to go through this process with such amazing people.

To my dog Maverick, who happily woke me up early to write, even if it was for an early cup of kibble. He was always willing to give me an extra nudge.

To Wiley Press staff, I would not have written this book if I had not been asked. I feel grateful for this opportunity and all that this process has taught me.

Introduction

Disclaimer: Please do not see this book as a replacement for therapy. Each individual is different in their experience and responses. If topics in this book trigger past events or worsen things, please contact a licensed professional in your area. I utilize information gained from many years of therapy, and I utilize skills I sometimes use in a therapeutic office, but please do not consider this book therapy. There are countless ways to work through work-related stress, and I am only scratching the surface in this book. Please expand your knowledge as it speaks to you as an individual.

I want to recognize that many indigenous healers utilized skills discussed in this book and others very effectively before the skills were rewritten and researched in a clinic setting. Thank you to all who came before me, both acknowledged and not, who paved the way for healing. We would not be here if it were not for everyone who came before us.

Introduction

CHAPTER 1

WHAT YOU CAN EXPECT FROM THIS BOOK

The field of veterinary medicine has some significant differences from other professions. These differences create different responses unique to veterinary medicine. While other healthcare professionals have some similar struggles, veterinary professionals are the only healthcare professionals working with animals. With the unique challenges of veterinary medicine, veterinary professionals' struggles with well-being have often been overlooked. Learning about risk factors and the reasons behind the well-being crisis can help you better understand why your system may be reacting in a certain way. You can you grow your resilient to the inherent risk of the field so that you can thrive as a veterinarian.

Emotions are like a little kid pulling on your pants leg when you are trying to talk to another adult. Sometimes, we finish what we are saying, ask what they want, and they say, "I forgot," and run off. Sometimes, they ask for a simple thing, and all is well. If we do not stop and ask those questions, they will start to throw tantrums and get louder and louder. In the same way, if we shove our emotions and never return to them, they begin to throw a tantrum and show up in ways that do not necessarily make sense. It is not always appropriate to respond to the toddler immediately. Sometimes we need to finish a conversation before checking in on them. This, too, is similar to emotions. It is impossible to cater to them at all times of the day, especially in a high-stress, fast-paced environment. It is okay and necessary sometimes to say, "Not right now, let me finish this, and I will get back to you." The most important part is actually checking in; otherwise, the emotions (and the kid) stop believing you.

In this book, we will explore the purpose of our emotions and reactions so that you can listen to them when needed. This insight will make the reactions feel less scary or broken and more accessible for change. We'll talk about what we can do to understand stress from a nervous system level so that you can nurture your nervous system and its natural reactions. Understanding why your body reacts the way it does to keep you safe gives you the power to manage the reaction. You can start to love your body system and its response instead of feeling broken or like it is tearing you down. Human kind has existed for many years, thanks to our nervous system and its reactions. I would love to keep it that way. As you start to understand your nervous system, you will also learn skills that you can use to nurture it, no matter how high the stress level is. You will learn how to communicate with your nervous system, not just your mind. This may feel counterintuitive to some, as you may have learned that managing thoughts makes emotions disappear. However, I am sure you have experienced times when, no matter how many skills you use to eliminate the feelings, they just won't go away. They are saying, "Hey dummy, you are in danger, listen to me." You are not listening, so they get louder.

Many of our reactions to situations are regulated by our body, more so than our brain. The communication pathways in our body are very complicated. The brain communicates to the body how to react, and the body communicates to the brain how to respond. When we focus solely on our super loud thoughts that seem factual, we miss a whole chunk of our reaction. We can tell our brain it is wrong all day long, but our body system stomps its feet and says, "No, you might die from this; listen to me!" Thoughts about situations are simply neurotransmitters firing, but they sometimes feel like cold, hard facts. An argument I often hear is, "Wait, are you saying my thoughts are not important?" I would like to clarify that your thoughts are very important. You worked hard to build facts into your brain and to form working thoughts. I am speaking of the idea that there is a big, complicated mess underneath the thoughts, making them hard to manage. Thoughts based on our studies are factual. Thoughts based on reactions may not be. Understanding, changing, and managing body reactions can be simpler than making significant changes in your life, changing your thoughts, or trying to snap out of it. Notice how I said simpler, not simple. None of this stuff is easy.

While I acknowledge some structures and culture within the field that make well-being more challenging to obtain, the primary focus of this book will be on your response to the current realities in the field. Stress is not just a response to what is around you; it is the interaction between you and the environment (Lecec-Tosevski et al., 2011). If you cannot change your environment, your best bet is to change how you respond to it. When large changes can be made, this allows you to see more clearly. Once you can ground and feel less emotional, I encourage you to fight for the changes you feel need to be made. You can do this through advocacy, education, and open conversations with those around you. I can assure you that these conversations will be more effective when emotions are at a manageable level. The emotions mimicking a toddler throwing a tantrum don't always communicate effectively.

HOW DOES THIS LOOK FOR ME?

My burnout story is one that almost anyone in any kind of healthcare setting can likely relate to in some way. I caught it early enough that it was not as dire as it could have been, but I was on the way. I was working for an agency that brought me up as a young therapist. I drank their Kool-Aid and thought that I was a top-notch therapist working for them. I was doing 30-minute sessions that were mostly paperwork. I enjoyed learning, and I could receive training for free as long as it fit within the clinic's values. I also struggled to apply the skills given the clinic dynamics and the short sessions.

Over time, I realized I wasn't the quality therapist I thought I was. I was told it was impostor syndrome and that if I read the script, I was doing well. I thought this was what therapy looked like. It was all I knew. I started taking my clients' stories home, and I would worry and dream about them. I mentioned this to people around me, who told me to stop taking it so personally. (No skills were given, just a simple, "Well, stop it.") I thought this was just part of being a therapist. I was told to take my lunches, and this would help. I also needed to get clinic hours and paperwork done, which sometimes required eating at my computer. I wasn't sure why I chose this career; it was not filling my cup. I started getting lazy and doing just enough to get by. This is outside of my values as well, but I got away with it, and looking back, I was trying to survive. The pay was something to be desired. I lived in what used to be a friend's closet to save on rent. When I spoke to others about the pay, they would often say, "I am not in it for the money," so I felt ashamed thinking I should be paid more.

I started feeling like I needed to work just to work. I gave up on what used to give me passion, thinking it must have been delusional. At some point, I was encouraged to write down what is important to me at a job. I believe it was a team-building activity meant to bring us all together. As I looked at what was important, I started to see my job with new eyes. I re-established my routine to fit into my value system and asked for things important to me, like longer sessions and clients wanting to work through their trauma. I still had to do the paperwork, but I was able to establish something that fit my needs and values. If I asked, this particular clinic was okay with making adjustments (to an extent). I developed a work life that fit closer to my values. It still wasn't perfect, but at least things had changed at some level. I eventually left that position feeling like they could no longer give me the growth I needed, but I did not leave the field, and I did not leave because of burnout. I look back and I appreciate what this job gave me as a young therapist.

It felt good to know that I worked through the burnout and established well-being, only leaving when it was the right time, not as a way to run away. I was less knowledgeable about the nervous system then, but when I look back, I can point out ways my nervous system fought for safety as I lived outside of my values. I can see how each employee's nervous system responded to each other, sometimes pulling each other down when everyone was discouraged. I can see that I nurtured my nervous system without even realizing it. I started working toward my needs instead of what was told to me.

As I write this book, I notice all the bodily reactions. My brain says, "Yes, you have all this important information, and it is important to write it down so that other people can apply it to their lives." However, I sometimes think people will label me a fraud (hello, impostor syndrome). I have thoughts about this being a big flop. I feel excited that many veterinarians and people in the veterinary field will read this book and find life-changing messages. My excitement feels similar to fear, leading to thoughts that I might not get done or meet requirements. I feel vulnerable that all these concepts rolling around in my head will be on paper, and I will have no control over who reads this. Basically, I feel all the feelings. My brain argues with the feels, but I still have them, no matter how much I tell them to disappear.

These responses lead to writer's block, procrastination, and a desire to run as far away from my computer as possible. I have even caught myself sitting at my computer, staring into space. I have no control over these reactions I speak about; they are just there, but I can gain control over what I do with them and how much I let them control me. If you read this, I can only assume I worked through my nervous system responses. I built safety in these hard tasks, which sometimes feel like they might kill me. I finished the book.

These similar responses continue to show up in my work as a therapist. Sometimes, my personal life drains so much energy that working takes my last bit of energy. I am very good at powering through when needed, which can catch up to me during busy parts of my life. Due to all of these factors, I had times when I did not show up to work at my best. I have felt disconnected from the people I worked with, going through the motions of the day. I have come home irritable or anxious, bringing the stress of the workday to my nondeserving loved ones. I had periods of my career when I was isolated from others, saying I was just too exhausted for other people. Luckily, I made it out of the difficult seasons alive. I have the skills to notice when I am not at my best before I become completely shut down or frantic.

My reactions to writing this book and difficult times in my career are not much different than how your body reacts to getting ready for work, being at work, leaving work, and just being in the profession of veterinary medicine. We are all using these skills together. I am a therapist. However, I am also fallible. Will writing this book kill me? Will your job kill you just by being your job? No, I can't imagine it will, but there are times when my body thinks it will.

I have rewritten my routines as a therapist, and most days, I genuinely like my job. I am better at what I do than ever, and I hope to be even better 10 years from now than I am today. My hiccups are learning experiences, and believe me, I learn a lot. I regularly apply skills I teach in order to keep my passion, enjoy my career, and do what I do well. Sometimes I use the skills more than others. Sometimes I need them more than others. The good news is that they're always in my back pocket. When I notice activation that does not fit the facts of the situation, I have practiced enough that they are easily accessible.

MY HOPE FOR YOU

When this book was proposed to me, it took me some time to decide that I wanted to write it. What ultimately brought me to sign the contract was the idea of providing skills and information in a different format to create accessibility to well-being. Suppose one person in a clinic can feel more like their authentic self. It can spread, and hopefully, one day the field of veterinary medicine can be a field where people thrive, live their love of animals, and no longer have to struggle in the career they chose and worked hard for. The culture of negativity and struggle can shift to one of passion and thriving. People no longer have to die in their misery; they can find a life worth living.

I have grand hopes for the field as a whole. I also have hope for you. I hope that you can apply the concepts of this book to understand yourself and your reactions and be the best veterinarian, employee, friend, partner, parent, handler, child, or whatever roles you have in your life you can be. You have the right to thrive as much as anyone else, and now is the time to do it.

I HOPE THAT YOU READ THIS BOOK AND:

- Gain acceptance of your whole self and your natural reaction to stress.

- Begin developing new patterns and routines that create safety, allowing your body to relax from the high-stress work environment that you are living in.

- Learn to use your reactions productively instead of feeling like they are "running the show."

- Allow space for the passion that brought you into this field and got you through veterinary school.

- Gain happiness, passion, identity, and connection to yourself, animals, others, and nature.

The stress of the veterinary world does not have to take over your life. I want this book to help you settle into the life you hoped for, even if you cannot label what that would look like now. You can create a sense that your profession feeds you and makes you a better person, rather than feeling like it is tearing you down and making other parts of your life more complicated than they have to be.

REFERENCE

Lecec-Tosevski, D., Vukovic, O. and Stepaniovic, J. (2011). 'Stress and personality', *Psychiatriki*, 22(4), pp. 290–297.

Utilizing This Book

While I am an expert in my field, only you are an expert in you. As you read this book, please know that none of this information fits 100% of people; we all have similar reactions, but there's still a difference in our experiences. We all have different amounts of neurotransmitters, we have all lived different lives, and we all have different families and cultures that we come from. This book is not designed to create shame when something does not apply to you or does not work. It is designed to provide information that helps you gain more awareness and safety in your body, ultimately leading to many veterinarians thriving. I offer a wide range of skills and a significant amount of information in this book. Please take what works for you and leave what does not.

This book is for people in all stages of burnout. If you are already burnt out and exhausted from your work in the veterinary field, this book can give your insight into ways to regain your passion for what you do. If you are inching toward burnout and are concerned about its impact on your well-being, this book provides strategies to restore resilience in the face of burnout. If you are not burnt out but terrified, you will be. This will guide you through resilience. If you are a practice manager wanting to grow a healthy culture of individuals who love their job, please share this information with your team.

THINGS THAT DO NOT WORK:

- Reading this book and hoping the information will sink in and "fix you" automatically. *It is easy to find information in the book interesting and read the content without applying the skills. Unfortunately, when it comes to well-being skills, practicing them is the only way for them to be effective.*

- Reading this book, and hoping the writer's motivation and hope will inspire you. *Hope only works for a little while and wears off quickly when it is not your own.*

- Trying skills with a sense of frantic "this must work perfectly and quickly" attitude. *Frantic skill use creates another layer of emotion that is difficult to work with. It is easy to fall into this trap because when you are struggling, you often wish you had felt better yesterday. It is hard to be patient. The problem is it can lead to hopelessness and shame. Allow for some patients when you can.*

- Trying to do the skills perfectly, just as they are described. *When you try to do these types of skills perfectly, it can distract you from actually doing the skill. You spend so much time planning for how you will perform and assessing your performance, you can lose track of the skill, and the assessment becomes skewed.*

THINGS THAT DO WORK:

- Reducing expectations and increasing curiosity. *This allows us to see what works for us and what does not. It removes the junk that comes from an "am I doing it right" attitude. It allows for a more pure use of skills.*

- Apply the skills as if they were a science experiment. You have a hypothesis of what will work, but you aren't quite sure how it will end up until you conduct the experiment. *When you shift your mindset from a "This must work for me" mindset to an "I wonder if this will work for me" mindset, you take away the pressure and are more likely to find the skills that work best for you.*

- Allow yourself to be creative and modify skills if you would like. *Again expert in the field, not in you. This is your life, and finding what works best for you and applying these concepts to your individual self is way more important than doing them right.*

- Try things even if you are skeptical that they will work. *You do not need an open mind for these skills to work. You might surprise yourself, or you might be correct, but at least give them a shot.*

- Embrace the weird. *Since many of us have learned to manage life with our thoughts, some of the stuff I discuss in the book may seem weird. It is common for someone to say, "I tried that thing you talked about to prove you wrong, and it worked." Please embrace the weird; if the other stuff is not working, you might as well. What's the worst that can happen? It doesn't work, you feel weird doing it, and you move on and try something else. That is not so bad.*

I acknowledge that these concepts are easier said than done. We will push up against that perfectionism that runs so rampant in the field. When perfectionism comes in, I encourage you to notice it and do the skill anyway. See what happens when you do something imperfect and it works.

ALLOW FOR THE SLOW

Many of the skills and concepts I discuss in this book seem simple. Sometimes, the simple skills don't seem like enough. Complex, big-change strategies are often too big for someone in a stressful environment. Small, simple-seeming skills usually allow more space for significant changes in your life. Just because something seems simple does not make it easy. Change is hard, no matter how you put it. Animals, including us, like routine and want to know what to expect. Even if what we expect is painful. When people finally seek help for change, they are usually sick of the pain and want things to work quickly. I can tell you right now that you should be skeptical of anything that says you should make significant changes, fast or easy. I have seen people make changes quickly, but they typically do not last. The body system cannot sustain significant, fast changes when shit hits the fan. Our system seeks the quickest, easiest way to get through challenging situations, which means it will default back to your current way of being, even if that way is destructive.

The good news is that slow is sustainable and over time becomes your norm, so that things can feel less burdensome. I can't tell you the exact amount of time you should spend grinding, but I can tell you that eventually, it will be less of a grind and more of a sustained change. As you use these simpler skills and they work, a positive reinforce forms in your brain, which means it starts to build a neuropathway for this method. Right now, your neuropathway communicates frantic, neurotic chaos if you are struggling. A new neuropathway is why you are here.

If you decide to change your routine completely tomorrow, it would be very stressful, and it would be easy for this change to fall flat. Many of us have seen this when we try to exercise, eat healthy, or meditate. If it takes too much time, or is too hard to achieve, it typically does not last. These small changes create space for you to make significant changes that have been proven to improve mental health naturally. There are only 24 hours in the day and way more expectations for what you "should" be doing than you likely have time for. This is why self-care can become a stress of its own. When managing stress effectively, you can also manage the stress of self-care.

When I discuss creating well-being in veterinary medicine, the answers I hear are often a top-down approach to change. The idea is that we need systematic change for change to happen. Policymakers, managers, and practice owners need to make changes for change to happen. I am not discrediting this idea at all. Some significant systemic changes can and need to be made. However, our first line of defense is in managing ourselves. When we can manage the current stress of the job and know how to regulate our body system to the stress of everyday life, things become more straightforward about how to work toward more significant changes at higher levels. When we work toward change in the same frantic, stressed-out system we live in, the change also feels frantic and stressed out. Education about well-being is still needed. There is more conversation about it, but we are not quite there. Some solutions are Band-Aids or artificial fixes to a huge problem. There is an expectation for burnout, compassion fatigue, and vicarious trauma. It is considered part of the job. This is not respectful to the people working their tails off in the day-to-day work of veterinary medicine. We need to start listening to each other and what we need for effective change to happen. This also means that we must be regulated and grounded to communicate those needs effectively. This means that we must be patient in our own healing in order to work toward healing the field as a whole. Waiting to ground yourself to work toward significant changes can also be frustrating. Patients is necessary here as well.

Some stressful parts of the job are necessary to serve the animals you are passionate about. This is hard to accept when we are talking about jobs. Animals are going to be animals; they will react, have a difficult diagnosis, and get old. Handlers will be handlers. I wish everyone in this world were kind and respectful to those around them and had a grasp on their emotional reactions, but I also can't control the whole community. Some parts of veterinary medicine require on-call work and long hours because of the nature of the animals that they treat. A level of acceptance is necessary with these unchangeable pieces of the job. With acceptance comes the ability to work with it instead of against it. This involves identifying skills, routines, and mindsets that nurture our system in such an environment instead of hoping it will change.

This book is not designed to answer all your questions about whether you should stay in the field or turn your life upside down and start something new. However, it does allow you to have a nervous system that can tolerate the natural stresses of the job so that you can decide fully if this is for you. Big questions and internal conflicts often become more apparent with a more grounded, safer system.

I cannot change the stressful nature of the field. I cannot change the challenges of veterinary school, the handler's treatment of veterinarians, or the system's struggles with well-being. I cannot change the constant life-changing and difficult decisions that present themselves in this field, and I can't even change your co-workers and colleagues, but I can create an avenue for changing your reaction to all of these things. Emotions are important. They communicate the necessary things to keep us safe. We will not change the fact that you have emotions, but we will teach you how to feel your emotions well.

PERSONALIZE YOUR GOALS

Just reading this book may be helpful for a short period of time. If you would like to make lasting effects, it is important to establish a goal for yourself as you read this book. Goals allow you to assess if the skills work for your own personal needs. Without goals or with a general, "I just want to feel better" goal, it can be difficult to see if any of the skills you are trying are working effectively. If I gave you a goal for the book, it also would not be effective. It would lack personalization and would fall short very quickly. To be as effective as possible in your process, it is important to establish your own goals. It is important to ensure your goal is small enough to be achievable and big enough to be challenging. If you need to, you can create a larger intention with steps for your goals.

When I was in my early 20s, I decided to do a triathlon for the first time. I enjoyed racing, and goals, so I thought it was a reasonable goal. Given my temperament at that time in my life, I did not want to make the smallest goal possible; I decided to do an olympic triathlon (1.5 K swim, 40 K bike, and 10 K run). I bought all kinds of equipment, read all kinds of books, developed a training plan, and began. I started with a master swim group. The instructor told me I was not a strong enough swimmer for the group. You see, I could always save myself, and could swim okay recreationally, but I never actually learned how to swim correctly. I took swim lessons and improved my form. I was a little off my training plan, but I felt like I could get back on track quickly. The weather got nicer, and it was time to bike. The thing is, I did not have a bike. That was an easy fix. I bought one and started biking to work, the perfect length for training. The water got warm enough to swim in a lake. People told me it was different from a pool, and I didn't believe them. It turns out that when I put my face down with googles on in a lake, I had unexplainable panic attacks (something I have never experienced before). I tried to use the skills I teach my clients, but I needed to stand and I could not touch the bottom. The whole thing was a disaster. I still had running, so I felt like I was doing well. I had an injury in my running. The defeat started to set in. I was doing half as well as I thought I was in my training. It was finally time to reduce my sign-up to a sprint triathlon (half the distance). I struggled with my decision. It made me feel like I am not good enough. Jump ahead to race day. I was so nervous, my stomach was in knots. I started the swim (not having conquered my anxiety). I was so anxious I had to have this nice lady in a pink kayak follow me the whole way. The lady in the pink kayak was my savior. She tried to explain to me that the water does not get deeper than 6 ft, but it didn't work. I made it through the race, swimming for small distances before she saved me. I was the last out of the water (except for a man who had vision problems and got lost along the way). I cried, but I kept going. Time for biking. After the race, my partner informed me that my bike tire was flat. No wonder it felt so difficult, and I went so slowly. I got to the transition from bike to run. I cried again. This time I am not quite sure why, I cried, it just came. On to the running portion. I had to walk a decent amount and was in pain from the injury I had during training. I crossed the finish line with someone who was throwing up as they passed. My cheering squad celebrated my achievement. I cried again. I looked back on my race and felt like a failure. It took me a long time to see the achievements in the race. Looking back, I realized I had set an unachievable goal and lacked smaller, achievable goals along the way. Life kept happening, and instead of acknowledging my setbacks, I simply felt like a failure. If I had set a flexible intention for the Olympic triathlon with small goals along the way, I could have noticed my accomplishments, and there were many. My intention could have shifted, and I could have celebrated crossing the finish line despite all kinds of adversity, rather than feeling like a failure.

This race is a great symbol for building resilience and recovery from well-being. We often make goals that are not achievable. We feel like a failure when we have to take a few steps back because of adversity instead of acknowledging accomplishments along the way. We set goals so big that they are debilitating. We forget to define the steps along the way. We purchase the equipment and develop a training plan without knowing what to expect, and we don't allow for flexibility as we learn along the way. If we set smaller goals that build on each other, we allow for a greater amount of flexibility. You can see in Figure 2.1 that when we focus on smaller steps in each step we are more likely to reach our intention. We feel accomplished along the way, and we often reach a point where we feel like we've met our intention, even if it shifts. As you can see in the figure, the goals can be like stair steps. Sometimes you may need to add a step as you go along. I didn't include buying a bike as a step, but adding it likely was effective as I went along. I probably also could have added overcoming anxiety in open water to the mix, but I did not know that when I made my plan. Instead, I felt defeated and struggled to know my accomplishments. When you look at change from this perspective, you allow space for curiosity along the way, shifting and changing as you gain more knowledge.

EXERCISE 2.1 | Establish your goals

1. Make a list of all the things you would be doing if your life were what you would like it to be. This list can be as ridiculous as you would like. I like to call this the "word vomit" part. If it comes to your head, write it out, no matter how absurd it is.

2. Go through and circle 1–5 that are reasonably achievable.

3. Is there a theme? If so, write it as your intention. If not, you can have two intentions.

4. Write about the smaller steps you will take to get to your intention.

5. Set a reminder on your calendar to revisit this goal sheet in 2 weeks. (if that feels too long, feel free to make it 1—this is your journey, make it personal)

6. Check in with your goals. Do the goals and intentions still apply? Sometimes, as we make changes in our lives, our goals shift and no longer apply. Does the next step feel too far away? Do you feel paralyzed in any way? If so, add more steps. Sometimes, we look back and cannot even remember who the person was who made those goals. We are farther along than we ever imagined. We've outgrown that person, and it's hard to believe we were that naive. Adjust as needed.

7. As you review, write down what is working for you. It can be easy to forget what works when life gets tough. Have this list handy for difficult times.

8. Repeat 1–5 as often as you would like to check in with yourself.

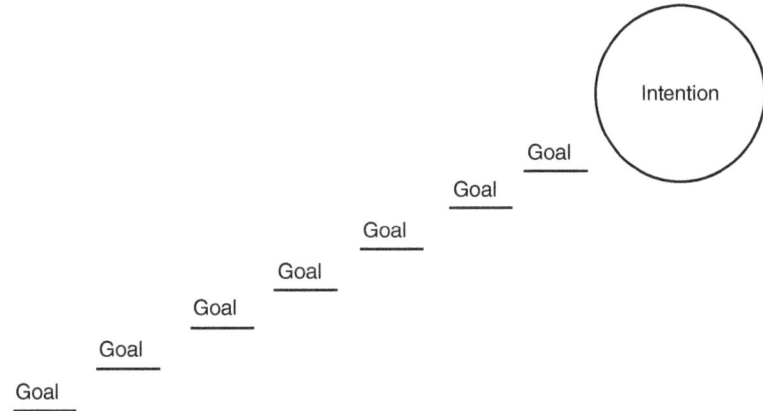

FIGURE 2.1 Allowing a goal to be each step of the way leading up to the intention allows for realistic and flexible goal making.

SUPPLEMENTAL JOURNALING

Due to the large amount of information provided in this book and the need to personalize it to fit your personal needs, I have included food for thought journal topics throughout the book. You can use these topics to solidify what you learn on your own. Even if you do not choose to use these, I recommend having some sort of ritual to help you digest the information. Some people struggle to identify with writing. You can modify this exercise through free-flow art, formal journaling that is legible and can be reread if desired, creative writing, such as poetry, or verbal processing with a trusted colleague. You may even dictate something to your phone, so that it can be less organized than talking with a colleague. Try a few ways to see what is best for you (Lindquist, Tracy, and Snyder, 2018).

While I recommend free-flow journaling, any method you use for journaling is a great way to connect your conscious thoughts with your subconscious thoughts (Lindquist, Tracy, and Snyder, 2018). Our thoughts often bounce around our heads like a bouncy ball in a small room; it is hard to catch and make sense of them. Free-flow journaling allows us to organize our thoughts, opening the door to let the bouncing ball roll out, letting the ideas flow so that we can see them more clearly. People do not need a fancy pen and notebook for journaling. Knowing that the written information will be thrown away or stored in a place only the writer can see allows you to be honest in your journaling activity. Knowing someone may read it and judge you or make assumptions allows for a spontaneous censor to appear, limiting the reflections that can be made (Lindquist, Tracy, and Snyder, 2018).

Free-flow journaling is the act of just writing whatever comes into your head. I sometimes call it "word vomit journaling." This is different than note-taking in that it doesn't have to make sense, nor should it. You will never reread it; it is just a product of your train of thought. I recommend practicing free-flow journaling with a pen and paper, rather than a keyboard, as I find something very powerful about the act of writing using pen and paper. However, many people utilize a keyboard and computer screen and have great success. While writing, your mind can jump from topic to topic or stay focused. The key to this practice is to let it happen without expectation. Pull out a piece of paper after you read a section of the book, while your mind is trying to put all the pieces together. This can be anything from a nice fancy notebook to the brown paper bag that your take-out meal came in, and everything in between. Set a timer for 3–7 minutes. A defined amount of time is essential, because if you have nothing else to say, I recommend writing, "I have nothing else to say." What happens as you continue writing can be fascinating. If you have a ton to say, you can fill up multiple pages, and it may or may not be productive. Now, just write. Sentences might not be complete; words might not be legible; just write whatever pops into your head for the allotted time. If you think the exercise is stupid, write, "This is stupid." If you are confused, write "I am confused." I mean this literally when I say to write whatever pops into your head.

Extra Credit: Do the same with your less dominant hand. When your timer goes off, switch hands. For some, like me, you might barely be able to make out letters on this one, but it can be very interesting to see what opposing thoughts come up as you write with your opposing hand. This occurs because the right side of the brain is more active when using the left hand, and the left side of the brain is more active when using the right hand (Boyraz et al., 2021). When under stress, our body often functions more dominantly from one side of the brain. This is why it is difficult to see the whole picture of a situation when under stress. This exercise allows you to open both sides of the brain and see the whole picture.

Now stop and reflect. If you are a list person, create a brief list of what you consider essential about your writing. The reflection part can take less than a minute; it is simply a step to regroup and decide what is important about your task:

Figure 2.2 shows an example of a free-flow journal entry using opposing hands. Notice how it is not legible, does not make sense, and is messy as all get out. Yep, that's what you are looking for. This figure portrays a 10-minute free-flow writing exercise about procrastinating cleaning my house. Five minutes were spent using my right hand, which is my dominant hand, and 5 minutes were spent using my left hand. Thirty seconds were used to remind myself of insights. I used a piece of paper that my kids left lying around, ripped and crinkled. Notice how imperfect this is; however, it did remind me that I need to be kinder to myself, set up organized time for my tasks, and ground myself because when I am frantic, nothing gets done. Yes, I did clean my house that day. It doesn't always happen like that.

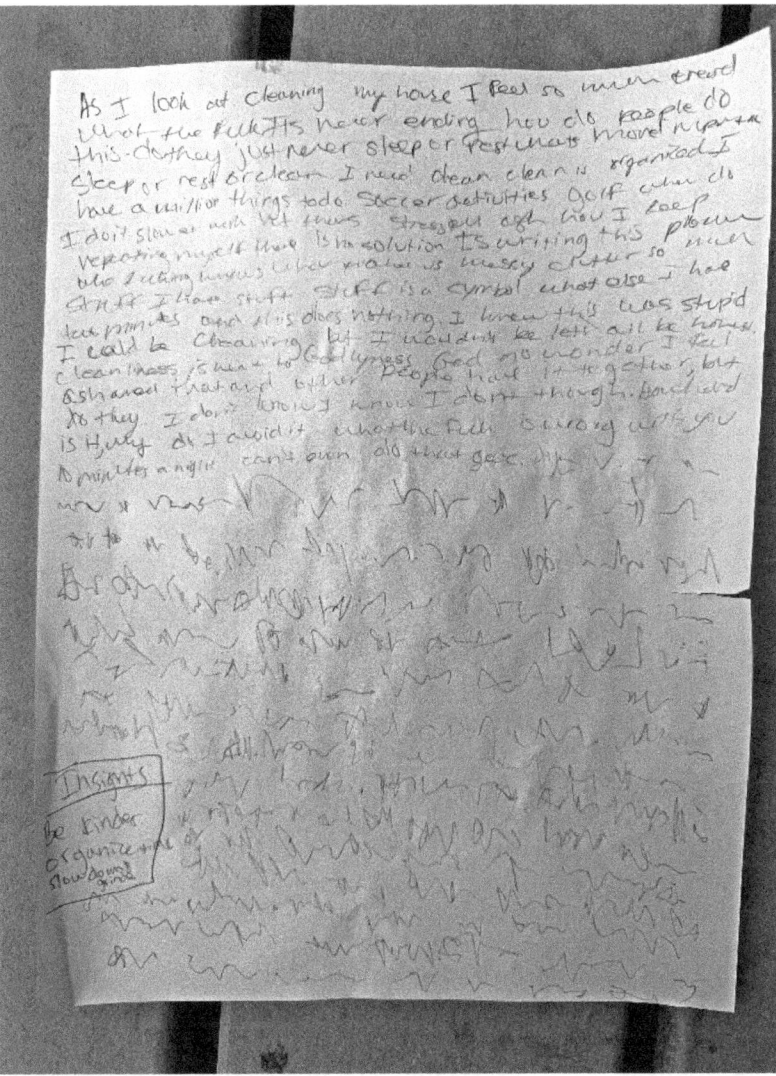

FIGURE 2.2 Example of free-flow journaling using opposing hands.

When doing this exercise with groups of people, I have received interesting feedback. Some people ask me if they have a mental health diagnosis they do not know about because one hand's responses are so wildly different than the other. (The answer is no, this exercise allows both sides of the brain to have an opinion, which they don't always do.) People have asked me what is wrong with them because they are all over the place. (The answer is nothing; our brains are often all over the place. Doing this regularly helps organize the all over the place.) People also complain that it makes their hands hurt. We do not use manuscripts as much as we used to, so some people's hand muscles struggle to get back into extended periods of handwriting. Shortening the time if your hand starts to cramp and work up to 5-minute increments. You can also stretch or rub your hand and return to writing if needed. This is not meant to be torture; do what you need. People have asked me how often one should do this. I personally use this exercise when I am stuck on something I can't quite make sense of. I know people who do it every night or every morning. How regularly you do this is totally up to you.

FOOD FOR THOUGHT JOURNAL TOPIC:

- What do you think about this whole journaling thing?

- What would get in the way of you trying it out?

- Try a free-flow journal without a topic and see how it goes for you to write whatever is on your mind at this moment.

CREATE A NEW ROUTINE

When we discuss improving well-being, we refer to shaking up habits that have become routine. Cynicism, negativity, and thoughts about hating your job can become a routine, just as the day-to-day grind can become mundane and a habit. This is why we sometimes go into autopilot mode and go through motions without even thinking about it. In graduate school, I had a professor create challenges for me to complete once a week. The first was to put your pants on the opposite way. If you are used to putting your left leg in first, try putting your right leg in or vice versa. The next step was to commute to school and work in a direction different from what you are used to. The third was to change up your nightly routine. If you brush your teeth first, try washing your face first (etc.) I struggled with this assignment. My mid-20s self was stuck on autopilot in life. I often would get dressed and think, "Oh shoot, I was supposed to do that thing." Or I would be halfway to work and realize I planned to go a different way but didn't. Not only did I forget to do it, but even when I reminded myself right before doing the tasks, I tripped and fell while putting on my pants, I got lost on the way to school, and I was discombobulated getting ready for bed.

This exercise aimed to teach us that changing routines can open our eyes to a new way of thinking, but I learned so much more about routines in the process. While changing routines can create awareness and mindfulness, shaking things up enough to make you think twice, it is also challenging on many levels. People typically don't choose to disregard new skills and tasks because they do not want to. It is usually because the autopilot kicks in, and it is difficult to remember. I recognize that changing routines is more than just a set-it-and-forget-it skill. It is so much more than this. I have now successfully attempted these challenges and continued to learn the difficulties of changing routines. This simple exercise, which was intended to teach me a minimal lesson that changing routine can allow you to notice other parts of your life that you ignore, taught me so much more. Change has stumbles in it. Mistakes will be made when you are stepping out of what you know right now, but in the long run, you can reset your thinking and slow down just enough to make the changes that really matter. I also learned that resilience is not a result of a lack of want or trying; it is often just a well-grooved routine.

You may have good intentions to try something, but forget, like I did the first time I tried this challenge. That is okay; it tells you that it is a challenging task. If you forget, try finding an alternative way to remind yourself. If you feel frozen in doing the task, break it down into smaller tasks and see if the smaller tasks are easier to accomplish. You may stumble through as you try out new things. That's okay. Give yourself space to try a few things and explore how this information resonates with you. Give yourself grace as you change your routine and try new skills and ways of thinking.

Changing routines can involve the things I listed above (putting your pant legs on differently, going a different direction to work, or changing your nightly routine) or others, such as sitting in a different chair when you eat, rearranging furniture, or anything that shakes up the autopilot. The goal is to make our brains work harder, creating space for new skills, tasks, or mindsets.

While changing routines can be beneficial, adding new ones can be just as helpful. This can be just as challenging as changing routine. We are creatures of habit. The exercise below can help you remember when creating new routines or modifying existing ones. Remembering is often the hardest part of change.

EXERCISE 2.2	Creating a cue

1. Think of a cue that will help remind you to cater to your well-being. When deciding on a cue, think of something you do all day long, so you do not forget the challenge. If you miss it once or twice, that's fine; even doing it sometimes is better than you were doing before. *Ideas of cues can include crossing door thresholds, drinking water, opening your email, driving signals like stoplights, or going to the bathroom.*

2. When the cue presents itself, tell yourself "This is my cue." These steps help us become accustomed to using the cue.

3. Pick something you learned from this book and apply it to this cue.

4. At the end of the day, check in to see if you are following through. If you are not, try a different cure. You can try out many cues and decide which works best for you. Make sure it is a cue you see or do several times a day.

Example: I decide my cue will be to check in whenever I cross a certain door threshold in my office. The visual of the door threshold reminds me, "Hey, remember you were going to try something new right now." I just read the section about the nervous system last night and decided to check in and see how my nervous system is reacting right now. As I walk to my next task, I check in. I notice that I am a little anxious and frantic, and I attribute this to a fight-or-flight response. I move on until I cross this threshold again.

DO A WALK THROUGH

In this section, we will discuss a visualization exercise. Some people can visualize, and some cannot. If you are a visualizer, visualize; if you cannot, just think about the concept and try to feel the emotions.

You may have noticed that when someone gives us a task to try out, it is easy to get excited at the moment about the new skill that may change our lives, but when push comes to shove, it gets lost in the shuffle of life. The reason this happens is that under stress, the body defers to the easiest mode of coping. Unfortunately, many times the easiest way to cope in the short term is the least effective way to cope. When we learn new skills, they do not come easily, and the brain tends to push them aside. Doing a walk through creates a neuropathway that tells the brain that it has done the skill before. The more you practice it, the more likely it is to get into the quick and easy skills you can access during stress. Since veterinary medicine has many layers of stress, you may not have time to practice the skill under low or no-stress situations. If you walk through the stress and use the skills when they are not actually happening, you may have a better chance of using them when things get busy.

Changing routines in the hubbub of day-to-day life is challenging. We often fall into autopilot or work mode and forget everything except the task at hand. If you have ever played a sport or an instrument or participated in a challenging task that needs practice, you may know that practice tends to be more mechanical, and the actual game, production, or concert has more flow. The same can be true for veterinary school. When you first learn the skill, you think through every step of the way, which is often very mechanical; however, the 500th time you do this skill, there is an added flow to the task. In this exercise, you will be in a more mechanical practice mode, making it more likely that you will use it when you get into a flow state.

Doing a walk through also helps us notice potential barriers before they arise. When we are moving quickly during the day, as we often do, we frequently fail to see what gets in the way of our follow-through. We start to feel shame for not following through, without acknowledging what may have gotten in the way. By practicing our plan visually, we can slow down the process so that we can notice the barriers, and plan around them making it more likely for us to follow-through.

EXERCISE 2.3 | Do a walk through

---

1. Pick a time when you have just a few minutes. Maybe before you go to sleep, when you first wake up, or on the car ride home.

2. Walk yourself through your day in as much detail as possible. Insert the skill or concept you want to be curious about throughout the day. If you added a cue, watch yourself doing this as the cue presents itself. This is a practice round for applying the skills and concepts. You can write this out, speak it in detail, or visualize it, but the most important part is giving as much detail as possible. *Do not overlook the difficult emotions you may feel throughout your day; this is about being realistic, not idealistic.*

3. Notice how it feels to apply the concepts learned during these difficult emotions. If you notice a resistance or difficulty using the skill in the visualization, create some curiosity around the place you see the struggle. The nice thing about this is that we can explore the parts that make it hard before the outside world becomes difficult. Here are some examples of struggles you may have and how you could address them.

   a. You are confused by the skill. *It can be difficult to do a skill you don't understand.* *Go back and read the section of the book. If it still does not make sense to you, try this with a skill that does make more sense.*

   b. If it feels too big (even if it is a simple skill logically), something in your body makes it seem overwhelming. *Make it smaller. If you are visualizing taking full breaths, start by exhaling. Make it as small as necessary to complete the exercise. Once this becomes more natural, you can increase the difficulty.*

   c. You feel some resistance to the new skill. *Think through this more mechanically. Notice the "I don't wanna" and see if there is a way to argue with it and do it anyway.*

   d. Secondary gain. *This is a difficult one because none of us wants to admit that we get secondary gain from something ineffective or even destructive. If we are trying to stop a behavior with the skill, there may be resistance because we are getting some benefits. For instance, family or clinic dynamics may be influenced by the behavior; people may give you more attention, which can allow you to be seen, even if it is in a negative light. Explore whether you are receiving any secondary gain that makes it difficult to change.*

I did not make this up. Many Olympians engage in this practice before competing in their sport, a strategy that dates back to the 1950s. They picture themselves going through the act in the way they hope to do it. This inserts the concept into the neuropathway, and your brain believes you have done the task before, making it more likely that you will accidentally think about it when you get into the day's groove.

Suinn and Richardson (1971) noticed this exercise and applied it in a similar way to how muscles contract and relax to facilitate movement. He saw that if something is very tense, adding some relaxation can allow it to flow more easily. Encouraging people to practice relaxation or a sense of success while visualizing stress or difficult situations appears to have the same effect.

EXERCISE 2.4	Contrasting emotions walk through

1. Bring to mind a time when you felt relaxed or successful. Picture yourself in this place as detailed as you possibly can.

2. Notice where and how you feel this feeling in your body. Hold this sensation for a moment.

3. Now bring up the stress of the day again, this time while holding the feeling of relaxation in your body.

4. Notice that the stress and the relaxation may argue with each other. Continue to hold them together in this visualization.

5. Allow both sensations to coexist. If they argue and go back and forth, allow them to. Ideally, they will both be present at the same time; however, this is not always possible when first practicing this exercise.

You don't have to spend much time on this, or you can spend a considerable amount. If you are short on time, try to find a moment when you can do this while working on a different task. You can practice your run-through while you do the dishes, in the shower, or during your commute to work. Some may argue that it is better to do it meditatively and for a longer period of time. Yes, it is more effective to do it when you can do it fully without distraction and in large chunks of time. However, I have taught skills to many people and understand that if the task is too big or takes up too much time in a busy schedule, it will not get done. If you are unlikely to do it, it is better to do it distracted and not perfectly than not do it at all. Consider when you will actually carry this out and make that your plan. Any practice is practice. You can add to it as you are able. Eventually, you can work up to a full meditative visualization if that is something you would like to work toward.

DO WHAT WORKS FOR YOU

I say over and over again in this book, "Do what works for you?" or "Modify this as you need." How annoying is that? Shouldn't I just tell you what you should be doing and know it will work? No, every person is different. I am an expert in the field, but only you are an expert in you. Disc assessment, enneagram, Myers-Briggs, and other personality tests are popular for a reason. These types of evaluations can be beneficial in identifying your learning, coping, and communication styles. Part of a positive well-being is having access to your authentic self and trusting it. The problem is that, over time, we lose trust in ourselves and feel like we are broken or have no insight. These assessments can start the ball rolling if you need a foundation for understanding who you are. You can also naturally build confidence in your authentic self by looking at skills with curiosity and wholeheartedly deciding what works best for you.

We are inundated with the way that we should be. The ideal way to be in order to gain organization, communicate, and approach life. I see articles everywhere teaching us how to block schedules, follow through on goals, and be a better, happier person. Sometimes, this information is helpful and allows us to shape our lives as we hope to. At other times, it creates shame and frustration because it is inauthentic, and we just can't do it. Trusting your core being and who you are, without all the extraneous stuff on top, allows you to sort through the should. Trusting yourself is difficult and comes with time, but it is well worth it.

The thing is, unless your authenticity fits a box, the box won't fit. As you read and explore in this book, I encourage you to explore what is authentically you. Does this skill or concept push on a value or trait of yours? If it does, is it a good push (challenges you to be better), or does it feel like it takes you out of who you are authentically? While journaling, ensure that you are not writing about what you should be writing or who you should be. Things can often be stressful because they are not authentically you, and you are forced to fit into a mold. Change is hard enough; we can at least take the should layer off of it. As you go through this book, allow yourself to be curious and let yourself find what works for you in each moment while also challenging your current habits and knowledge. Don't skip it just because you don't like it. Try it out, see how it works, then decide.

FOOD FOR THOUGHT JOURNAL TOPIC:

- What am I skeptical about as I start this book?

- What am I scared of as I start to make changes?

- How do I want this change to look for me?

- What are my shoulds?

REFERENCES

Boyraz, R. K. *et al.* (2021). 'A treatment-response comparison study of resting-state functional magnetic resonance imaging between standard treatment of SSRI and standard treatment of SSRI plus non-dominant handwriting task in patients with major depressive disorder', *Frontiers in Psychiatry*, 12, 698954. https://doi.org/10.3389/fpsyt.2021.698954.

Lindquist, R., Tracy, M. F. and Snyder, M. (2018) 'Journaling', in *Complementary and Alternative Therapies in Nursing*. New York: Springer Publishing Company, pp. 201–209.

Suinn, R. M. and Richardson, F. (1971). 'Anxiety management training: A nonspecific behavior therapy program for anxiety control', *Behavior Therapy*, 2(4), pp. 498–510. https://doi.org/10.1016/S0005-7894(71)80096-5.

Special Populations

As I mentioned, we are all human and have personal struggles. Most people have personal struggles outside of their careers in the field of veterinary medicine. Some people's stressors stem from how their brain functions, their perspective on the world, and their background. When a person's brain functions differently from the social norm, or they feel different due to their appearance, it can exacerbate the natural stressors of the job. Feeling "othered" or like you are not accepted by those around creates added pressure to fit in and conform. It is important to remember that some people struggle differently from others. As you begin to support each other from a nervous system perspective, give some space to the lived experience of others. Be mindful of how the language you use can influence those around you. If someone says they are offended by a way you say something, it can be a place to learn and grow. It is easy to become defensive, but acknowledging this can help us move from defensiveness to openness. I may say something in a way that is difficult for some as they read this book. I encourage you to reach out and let me know.

It is essential to acknowledge and raise awareness about a few populations that are often overlooked in discussions of veterinary medicine, so that we can all be mindful of their needs. While I am speaking specifically to a few populations, this is not assuming that these are the only populations who suffer or feel excluded.

NEURODIVERSITY

Neurodiversity is used to describe the way all brains function differently, and implies there is no correct way to learn; however, there are many instances where traditional education and social norms do not conform to all brains. The term "nerodiverse" has been used to describe a person whose brain does not conform to the general cultural norms around them. There is a long list of diagnoses that fall under the category of neurodiversity, such as Autism Spectrum Disorder, Attention Deficit Hyperactivity Disorder, and Dyslexia. For the sake of this book, I will not focus on the diagnosis as much as some learning types that may struggle in the field. Because all brains function differently, I may miss something; however, I want to emphasize that traditional medicine and social norms can be especially challenging for specific individuals.

Regardless of how your brain interprets the environment around you, we are all humans reacting to our surroundings and trying to stay safe. For a neurotypical person (someone whose brains fit into the norms of the culture around them), workplace structures, school, and day-to-day tasks can feel like they are set up to help people succeed. When someone is less successful, it is because they are not working hard enough or not smart enough to understand the concepts. However, certain people may thrive within a modified structure that accommodates their brains. Allowing for flexibility with accommodations can create a space where people can feel more accepted and can use their strengths in a way that they can thrive (Quigley *et al.*, 2024). When people have not felt like they can conform in other aspects of life, such as schooling, it can translate into the workplace when we do not create space for people to have their needs met. If accommodations are not met, people may continue to feel a sense of lack of acceptance. Mixed with the everyday stressors of veterinary medicine, this can be detrimental to mental health. Covering up what you have interpreted as flawed and working hard to conform is exhausting.

A person who falls into the category of neurodivergence is more likely to be depressed and anxious, and they have a high suicide risk (Smits, 2022). People learn to conform as much as possible to make it through, leading to self-silencing. Feeling different from those around you is uncomfortable. People learn to mask their emotions or struggle to maintain the status quo (Syharat *et al.*, 2023). People who do not feel like they belong to the social structure and attempt to conform can feel isolated and lonely when their brains are not taken into consideration. The struggle becomes more difficult as they may be hesitant to speak out due to this tendency to conform. This all leads to the high levels of depression and anxiety. Each person has a different level of empathy; however, veterinarians are expected to have a specific level of empathy for those around them.

Handlers expect veterinarians to have empathy for them, not just the animals. However, some people's brains naturally empathize more with animals than with humans. We cannot decide how much genuine empathy we have; our genes determine our empathic abilities, which may differ among people or animals (Aurélien *et al.*, 2021). I would guess that many veterinarians would fall into the category of empathizing heavily with animals; however, they are also interacting daily with other humans, such as handlers and colleagues, who crave empathy. There are many theories about why one may show more empathy toward animals than humans, maybe because animals are more transparent about their emotions. When humans are masking, you may get a sense of one emotion when they are actually showing another. Some say it may be because animals do not give corrective feedback when people are wrong or misinterpret an interaction (Aurélien *et al.*, 2021). Whatever the reason, it makes sense to me that someone who has received negative feedback about their interactions may become anxious, making it even more depleting in a world where empathy is expected from others. I am not sure we can change all of society's expectations for empathy; however, understanding each other's strengths as well as struggles can allow us to support each other in our day-to-day work.

All the factors that contribute to feeling different can form a vicious cycle that can be difficult for people to endure. Stress can make it hard to communicate, and communication can make it stressful. A person who naturally shows less human empathy may be less likely to engage in niceties and small talk during their conversation. This is interpreted as cold and unkind. The person may now feel debilitated by the natural struggle and increased stress related to interactions with others.

Some neurodiversity individuals struggle with feeling overloaded by sensory stimulation. Phone ringing, people talking, and beeping machines may create anxiety and make it difficult to think (Smits *et al.*, 2023). While reducing high stimulation is sometimes possible, it is not always feasible when working in the veterinary field. Additionally, some individuals' brains function more effectively within a predictable environment and may struggle with unpredictability (Smits *et al.*, 2023). This can be very difficult in a high-stress veterinary clinic or among colleagues who may be less predictable. The added stress of struggling with the unpredictable can create a frantic or freeze response, which gets in the way of completing tasks.

Sometimes, a job can be modified to accommodate the needs of someone who is feeling additional environmental stress. Some factors in the field cannot fully accommodate the neurodivergent brain, but supporting someone overloaded by these environmental stressors can be very important in allowing them to work in the best way possible. Instead of criticizing someone for not doing their job well, it can be received better when telling someone what they can do differently to improve their performance. It is also important to acknowledge the needs of the people around you and work with them to support them in your clinic. Even if it feels like someone should know what they can do, presenting constructive feedback with detail is essential to ensure that someone does not feel attacked. Allowing space for people to ask for what they need in a nonjudgmental manner is a great way to create a safe space for all types of individuals.

Neurodiverse people may also have traits like hyper focus, detail-oriented, pattern recognition, and detailed problem-solving, which may be beneficial within veterinary medicine (Smits *et al.,* 2023). With increased empathy toward animals, people will likely be able to interpret their pain and connect in a different way, which will help with the treatment of the animal. Someone detail-oriented may be able to catch something that another provider may miss. While someone who sees the big picture more than the details may see something, the detail-oriented person may miss. This is why it is essential to notice the strengths that come with our natural tendencies and work together with all different types so that the clinic and the field can function at their best.

Whether you are a practice owner, colleague, or support staff, it is important that we support people no matter which way their brain works. When we try to cover up people's deficits, it can communicate that the person is wrong or broken, leading to increased well-being struggles. When we acknowledge people's strengths and needs, they often work more efficiently and increase their well-being (Smits, 2022). While this is true for all workers, it is especially true for people who have been mistreated due to their differences. People naturally magnify their deficits when they have been bullied for them. By magnifying strengths, people can naturally see a larger picture of their skills and ultimately utilize more of their strengths in the workplace, making them a more valuable employee.

If you are someone who has struggled in the ways mentioned or a different type of neurodivergence, you are not alone, and you are not doomed. There are many ways to break the cycles and gain confidence in yourself. Even though a feeling of being "othered" can add additional stress to an already stressful world, your brain has likely served you in some way. While I can acknowledge the struggles of being in a marginalized population, I do not believe these to be a deficit. As you become more in tune with how your brain works, you will be able to see your strengths in a greater light. I hope that you can create a space where neurodiversity traits can be utilized without requiring them to be masked. This will enable you to manage the additional stress while learning to enjoy yourself for who you are.

My goal is to write this book in a way that appeals to a wide range of readers whose brains are working differently. Some people will be able to use visualization experiences, while others will not. Some people will delve into the skills discussed with a great deal of detail, while others will apply them in a broad, big-picture way. Please keep in mind what works best for you as you explore the concepts in this book. If you are reading as a group, please keep in mind that the concepts will resonate differently with each person who is reading the book. Whether you are reading this book, supporting one another in the workplace, or leading a team, please keep in mind that people think and thrive differently. This flexibility provides a safe space for all, regardless of how their brains function.

DIVERSITY AND INCLUSION

I identify as a white, sic, middle-class, heterosexual female. I understand and recognize the privileges and flaws associated with these identities. I also want to acknowledge that many people reading this book may identify in a less privileged way. Populations that tend toward marginalization have more significant struggles with well-being. In this book, we will explore why the amount of stress in one's life can accumulate, making it larger and more challenging to manage. When one experiences the anxiety of feeling different from those around them, persecution (intentional or unintentional), or having to prove themselves at a greater level because of their race, gender, or identity, an extra layer of stress is added to their well-being.

In addition, generational trauma created from generations of prosecution can lead to a fear and stress level that may be higher for those coming from this background. The person may know where this anxiety is coming from, or may be confused, not knowing it came from generations of suffering. One may feel extra pressure or may feel like they must prove to people who see them as flawed and wrong. They may feel like a symbol of all people within their identity, adding extra pressure to perform to perfection. A feeling of being unaccepted can increase the need to work hard and perform tasks better than their counterparts. In addition to the unspoken pressure that often comes with being a part of a marginalized population, many people have experienced macroaggressions and outward aggressive behavior from others regarding their identity, which can create an increase in fear and a lack of safety.

People who feel they belong perform better, challenge themselves further, and are more resilient and satisfied (Burkhard *et al.*, 2022). The field of veterinary medicine has a high population of Caucasian individuals. In fact, in 2022, veterinary medicine was on the list of the top 33 whitest jobs in America (Burkhard *et al.*, 2022). People who are nonwhite often experience aggression, microaggressions and various responses that make people feel like they do not belong. People who are white passing (perceived as white when their heritage is different) may experience some privileges of a white person while also struggling with feeling misunderstood. They may also struggle with the generational oppression discussed above.

The field should work toward equity, where each person gets what they need to succeed, and inclusion, where people can feel welcome, comfortable, respected, valued, and supported, no matter what identity they hold. A place where people belong, which means that they can be authentically themselves, will well-being and productivity within the field. Diverse, welcoming teams perform better, focus on facts, and find better solutions (Burkhard *et al.*, 2022). This is not just for the comfort of the individual, but for the efficiency of the clinic and field as a whole.

I would also like to acknowledge that research can leave out certain groups of people. While I utilize a large amount of research in this book, it is important to acknowledge that if it does not apply to you, that is okay. Similarly, various skills are more suited to certain cultures than others. Allow space for your own personal values, culture, and needs.

VETERINARY PROFESSIONALS OUTSIDE OF DVM

While I often refer to veterinarians in this book, I acknowledge that many people work in veterinary offices and share similar concerns that extend beyond those of veterinarians who have earned a Doctorate of Veterinary Medicine (DMV). Veterinary assistants, veterinary nurses, veterinary technicians, and program managers often have smaller salaries, physically demanding work, and the same grumpy handlers. In addition to this, well-being rates are low, so they are likely dealing with an irritable veterinarian barking orders because their own nervous system is struggling. Skills in this book can be used by all levels of veterinary medicine, not just the DVMs. The clinic cannot run without the help of all the staff members within it. Various positions may have slightly different reasons for burnout, stress, or disconnection, but all positions are working in a high-stress environment prone to low well-being rates. The veterinarian of the clinic may have a high level of responsibility, but they cannot run without the help of others in the clinic. It is important to be mindful of the importance of all.

While a large amount of the current well-being research is done on DVMs in the veterinary field, others are likely struggling as well. Veterinary technicians also work long hours and struggle with value conflicts. They are more likely than the general population to engage in substance use, not engage in physical activity at work, and make poor nutritional choices. These workers are often forgotten when we discuss the struggles in veterinary medicine, and they often get the brunt of everyone's struggle with well-being. Sometimes, they are considered to be the grunt workers who are expected to do the dirty work; this does not feel good when you work hard to gain the expertise that you have (Fong and Kim, 2022). While veterinarians often have to manage angry handlers, technicians, and program managers are often the first point of contact for individuals unhappy with their care. Staff outside of DVM struggle with moral dilemmas as well. They are sometimes asked to assist with procedures they disagree with or that hold an emotional attachment, making it difficult for them. Character traits of neurosis apply to nonveterinary employees, and many of the stressors are similar. Of the nonclinical staff surveyed, 74% expressed symptoms of medium to high burnout rates in 2024. Nonclinical staff are suffering from psychological stress similar to their veterinarian counterparts, with 20% defining psychological distress, much higher than the 6% of the general population (Volk *et al.*, 2024).

As you read through this book, please acknowledge that managing your own nervous system is essential to the entire team, regardless of their position. When one person on the team is more regulated, the entire team benefits from the change. Please be aware of the staff's struggles, appreciate them, and listen to their concerns. All members of the veterinary team are struggling similarly, and all members of the teams are essential for the most effectiveness of the clinic and the field as a whole.

FOOD FOR THOUGHT JOURNALING:

1. Where do you see the field needing to grow to accommodate people who may feel marginalized?

2. Where can you grow toward providing equity?

3. Do equity conversations make you uncomfortable? Why? (This may not be obvious; it may become more clear as you write.)

REFERENCES

Aurélien, M., Grandgeorge, M. and Raymond, M. (2021). 'Exploring neurodiversity through biodiversity: empathy of people with autism towards living beings mostly differs for a single species, ours', *PsyArXiv*. https://doi.org/10.31234/osf.io/49qxj.

Burkhard, M. J., Dawkins, S., Knoblaugh, S. E. *et al.* (2022). 'Supporting diversity, equity, inclusion, and belonging to strengthen and position the veterinary profession for service, sustainability, excellence, and impact', *Journal of the American Veterinary Medical Association*, 260(11), pp. 1283–1290. https://doi.org/10.2460/javma.21.11.0477.

Fong, K. and Kim, S. (2022). 'Correlates of occupational stress on emotional and physical health in veterinary technicians', *The International Journal of Health, Wellness and Society*, 12(2), pp. 37–47. *Frontiers in Veterinary Science*, 10, 1064932.

Quigley, E., O'Hanlon, M., Brandes, M., Kennedy, R. and Gavin, B. (2024). 'Neurodiversity and third-level education: A lacuna between the strength-based paradigm shift and the lived experience', *Neurodiversity*, 2. https://doi.org/10.1177/27546330241277427.

Smits, F., Houdmont, J., Hill, B. and Pickles, K. (2023). 'Mental wellbeing and psychosocial working conditions of autistic veterinary surgeons in the UK', *Veterinary Record*, 193(8), e3311. https://doi.org/10.1002/vetr.3311.

Smits, F. (2022) *Autistic veterinary surgeons in the United Kingdom: Workplace stressors and mental wellbeing* [Master of Research Thesis, University of Nottingham]. Available at: http://eprints.nottingham.ac.uk/78517/1/14324658_Femke%20Smits_MRES%20thesis%20corrections.pdf

Syharat, C. M., Hain, A., Zaghi, A. E., Gabriel, R. and Berdanier, C. G. P. (2023). 'Experiences of neurodivergent students in graduate STEM programs', *Frontiers in Psychology*, 14, 1149068. https://doi.org/10.3389/fpsyg.2023.1149068.

Volk, J. O. *et al.* (2024). 'Merck Animal Health Veterinary Team study reveals factors associated with well-being, burnout, and mental health among nonveterinarian practice team members', *Journal of the American Veterinary Medical Association*, 262(10), pp. 1330–1337.

Mental Health and Well-Being

This section of the book will concentrate on what the struggles within the field are and why they exist. We will focus on both well-being struggles and mental health struggles. Due to the nature of the section, some individuals may experience validation. You may feel seen or like you are not alone in your struggles. After all, if I am writing a book about this, you must not be the only one suffering. Some may feel discouraged. With all of these facts stacked up against you, how could you possibly succeed in the field of veterinary medicine? Please note that we will also discuss how to manage the pain addressed in this portion of the book. I will not leave you hanging by your toenails, hoping it will get better. Anyway you experience this chapter, I encourage you to think about how the struggles in the field may apply to you and those around you. The more awareness we gain, the more likely we are to utilize the skills to build resilience and address struggles before they become too significant. By understanding the struggles within the field, we also gain the ability to recognize pain in those around us. The more we can support people in our community, the better the field becomes as a whole. If we build each other up, we all get to rise to the top together.

HOW MENTAL HEALTH AND WELL-BEING AFFECT THE FIELD OF VETERINARY MEDICINE

It is interesting to look at the contradictory research in the veterinary field. Ahha's white paper, "Stay Please," found that 30% of veterinarians plan to leave their current role, and half of those plan to leave the field altogether. In the 2024 study put out by Merk, they found that 20% of veterinarians experienced extreme psychological distress compared to 6.3% of the general population. At the same time, Merk states in their vet well-being presentation that 74% of veterinarians are satisfied with their careers. This leaves 25% of veterinarians unhappy with their career, which makes me wonder if this is a satisfactory number. It seems to me that the statistics are not wildly different, and both express that people want to leave due to psychological distress (Volk *et al.*, 2024). Looking at just those with DVM credentials, 44% want to quit before retirement, according to Ahha's paper "Stay, Please" (2024).

A struggle with well-being is costing the field of veterinary medicine large amounts of money. Neill *et al.*, (2022) found that burnout costs $104,000 per veterinarian due to turnover. Burnout is also directly correlated to fewer work hours, costing $56,000 per burnt-out veterinarian. According to Ahha, losing one employee costs a company 1.5–2×'s that person's salary within the year after finding another employee, training the employee, and allowing time to adapt to the new position.

Money is not the only consequence of the struggle in the field. People leaving the field is also leaving a strain on the field in relation to available services. Universities are trying to create more programming, lobbyists are fighting for or against lower-level veterinary positions, and board meetings are being held about how to survive the crisis related to the need for more people in the veterinary field.

Well-being and mental health also affect the quality of work within the field. People stay in the field, perform better, and support each other when they have the energy to do so. People who have lower levels of depression, anxiety, stress, and burnout receive higher satisfaction rates from their customers (Campbell *et al.*, 2023). This is because the symptoms create barriers to quality work. People may struggle with the idea of giving up perfectionism, but a preoccupation with self-doubt will hinder their ability to concentrate (Campbell *et al.*, 2023). The brain would ruminate on ways that the person could mess up or ways they have messed up in the past, instead of focusing on the task at hand, which they are likely very capable of when able to concentrate. In addition, people in an anxious, frenzied state are more likely to describe their thinking as "fuzzy" and report an increase in being distracted. They are more likely to second-guess opinions and make less effective decisions when their confidence struggles. Burnout is associated with lower perceived safety at work, more mistakes, and lower quality of care. This is not only a well-being concern, but it is also a quality control concern within the field (Campbell *et al.*, 2023). People are not performing at their best when well-being scores are low.

When people are unhappy at work, it often presents as snappiness, a short fuse, tone changes, and being edgy with co-workers. I can only assume that this would create burnout in the co-worker you are snapping at, creating a ripple effect of ineffective care in a clinic. In addition, this snappiness may manifest as annoyance with everything and a tendency to point out annoyances to those around you. This creates a level of contagion with well-being struggles (Campbell *et al.*, 2023). This snappiness and short, frantic nature can also contribute to ineffective communication and not providing all the information. This could negatively impact the treatment the animal is receiving from the handler. Inadequate communication can also get in the way of the quality of care from staff who follow instructions to the best of their ability.

Customer service also suffers when mental health scores are high and well-being scores are low. With difficulty managing emotions that arise, struggles with communication, and apathy toward the work, it is challenging to create a quality customer service experience for the handlers. As customer service suffers, people are less likely to receive care when their animal is in need.

With a need for more veterinarians than ever before, it makes sense that there is a need for more schools, more positions, and more care for the animals. This takes a significant amount of time and money to facilitate. Improving the well-being of the veterinarians already in the field can produce a higher quality of care, improved retention, and an increase in people entering the field. This would reduce the loads of the current veterinarians in the field, save money in training new staff, and increase the effectiveness of the field at large. Training one staff member is said to cost a salary and a half of the current salary. If 30% of those in veterinary medicine want to leave the field, imagine the financial impact (American Animal Hospital Association, 2024).

While well-being is increasingly being discussed in more CE events, it remains hindered by beliefs that the problem does not exist. People continue to believe in a "pick yourself up by your bootstraps" approach that leaves the change up to the individual more than to the field itself. More efforts are being made to attract new professionals into the field, rather than retaining trained professionals who are struggling and may potentially leave due to their difficulties. Well-being is discussed in a surface-level way, encouraging people to take more breaks and set boundaries without changes to the field as a whole. While I genuinely hope you will make changes to improve your well-being and life, I also hope the field can thrive holistically. When people start helping themselves, the well-being around them changes, and people begin to notice them, too, and can thrive.

RESOURCES

American Animal Hospital Association (2024) *Stay, please: Veterinary medicine has a problem—it's losing good people at an unsustainable rate.* Available at: https://www.aaha.org

Campbell, M. *et al.* (2023). 'A qualitative study exploring the perceived effects of veterinarians' mental health on provision of care', *Frontiers in Veterinary Science*, 10, p. 1064932.

Neill, C. L., Hansen, C. R. and Salois, M. (2022). 'The economic cost of burnout in veterinary medicine', *Frontiers in Veterinary Science*, 9, 814104 https://doi.org/10.3389/fvets.2022.814104.

Volk, J. O. *et al.* (2024). 'Merck Animal Health Veterinary Team study reveals factors associated with well-being, burnout, and mental health among nonveterinarian practice team members', *Journal of the American Veterinary Medical Association*, 262(10), pp. 1330–1337.

Vulnerabilities

You chose to work in a very high-stress career. Maybe you knew this when you signed up for it, or realized it halfway through the veterinarian school grind that left you wondering what you were thinking. Either way, it is likely no surprise that 90% of veterinarians classify their work as stressful (Smith, Barcelos and Mills, 2023). The question is, do we have to accept this level of stress, or can we learn to make changes to manage it well? The nature of the career will probably not change. Large-scale decision-making will always be part of your job, handlers will always be under stress when interacting with you, and your love of animals will always drive you to work a little longer and a little longer. The difference can lie in how you manage the stress and your perceptions of yourself and others. I wish managing stress were a required course in the university setting. It would certainly make a difference in the field.

Many people trade career dreams throughout their lifetime, transitioning from being an astronaut to a teacher, and eventually to a social worker, accountant, or another field they land in. It is rare to find a person who "always knew they would be an accountant." However, veterinarians are often naturally drawn to animals and have wanted to pursue a career in veterinary medicine their whole lives. One study shows that 41% of veterinarians knew they wanted to be a veterinarian as long as they can remember. Only 5% of individuals decided to become a veterinarian after the age of 25 (Waitz-Kudla *et al.*, 2023). People often develop an identity around their jobs when it is included in their lifelong dreams and goals. This means when people question your work, they are not only threatening your career and well-being, but also something that is a part of you, something you stand for, part of your identity. It hurts more intensely when the job does not match your values because it is a part of who you are. This lifelong identity of veterinary medicine also comes with a feeling of being trapped. If someone knew they would be a veterinarian their whole life and fully identify with it, what does it mean if they do not like it? What other career could they possibly consider?

Research into the well-being of veterinary professionals has grown tremendously in the last 10 years. We have learned much about why well-being is suffering, and the job is stressful. Day-to-day career-related stressors such as long hours, conflict with handlers, high expectations of others, financial stressors, large amounts of moral distress, and routine euthanasia are consistently listed as difficulties faced by veterinarians. Combined with the new avenue of complaints in technology, we can also add cyberbullying to the stress of day-to-day veterinary work (Cooney and Kipperman, 2023; Hilton, Burke and Signal, 2023; Smits, 2022; Smith, Barcelos and Mills, 2023). None of the research says it is a laid-back, low-stress job, and there is no reason for people to struggle. In addition to the stressors directly related to the demands of day-to-day work, workplace culture is also a vulnerability factor to stress. Looking at the American Animal Hospital Association's white paper in 2018, people are generally dissatisfied because of low pay, low appreciation, a lack of career development, unproductive teamwork, and a lack of caring from leadership (American Animal Hospital Association, 2018, 2024). All of these factors point to workplace cultures. When a field has struggled for as long as veterinary medicine has, its managers and decision-makers have often lived within an unhealthy culture, making it challenging to create a healthy workplace culture designed to improve well-being. People in higher-level positions may be burned out or experiencing compassion fatigue, making it easier to focus on the money made rather than the person doing the work. The trickle-down of well-being is essential to treating well-being in the field. This may not be the fault of the decision-makers; it is simply what they know in the field.

The number one factor affecting workplace well-being is working hours, followed by the number of consultations one has in a day, time in surgery, and staying late. The research reports that other contributing factors include the number of breaks taken, time spent catching up on paperwork, and the number of walk-in appointments (Hilton, Burke and Signal, 2023). This highlights the fact that time is indeed a valuable commodity. When people's time is not valued, their well-being often suffers. Unfortunately, in the culture of veterinary medicine, it is expected to prioritize work time over other time. It is not uncommon for someone to plan to take a break "after they finish this one thing" and never actually take it until they realize they are exhausted, hungry, and fried. This practice is not only expected but sometimes encouraged. In addition, if you see a distressed animal in the grocery store or the parking lot, you will likely help that animal, no matter how exhausted you might be. Veterinarians generally join the field because they have a deep care and connection with animals. This love does not stop when leaving work. There is a strong value in working harder because you care. Boundaries become more difficult because if you see a struggling animal outside of work, you are likely to help them, not out of people pleasing or lacking boundaries, but simply because you care (Dickson, 2023). This caring and love is not a bad thing. It, in itself, does not create a struggle with well-being. The difficulty comes when it gets in the way of taking care of yourself. What made you expect to work yourself to the bone? It's hard to tell, but I would guess that it is linked to the high rate of neurotic personality traits and high performers that I speak about in the personality section of the book.

Unlike their human-serving counterparts, veterinarians are often faced with decisions about life and death. Their patients have shorter life spans than their human treating counterparts. The options for euthanasia are a part of veterinary work. A piece that human treating counterparts are not faced with. This is a relief for many veterinarians as they know they can help an animal in pain. However, there is an increased stress as people may euthanize early due to financial constraints or may choose not to euthanize due to their attachment, creating an increase in suffering for the animal (Dickson, 2023). The decision is ultimately up to the handler, creating little space for your own morals and values to play a part in the decision. Euthanasia can come with both positive and negative experiences. While one may be relieved that the animal is no longer suffering, there is a large amount of mental health struggle that comes with it as well. You are still sitting with grieving handlers and may even grieve yourself. Thoughts about mortality may become prevalent, and views on death may change when it is witnessed often.

Research shows that 68% of small animal veterinarians have experienced regret about euthanasia, 84% have experienced sadness following euthanasia, and 59% experience guilt around euthanasia (Cooney and Kimperman, 2023). These statistics only speak to the people admitting the difficulty of euthanasia. I have met many veterinarians who struggle to admit to the difficult parts of euthanasia for fear of being judged by others. The research does not state that every euthanasia experience is challenging or that you must struggle with euthanasia. It simply states that some may be hard, and it is difficult to treat your sadness when it is taboo to acknowledge the difficulty.

Grief needs to be processed, which, unfortunately, takes time. However, there is no time to process it in a fast-paced environment such as veterinary medicine. Grief does not always mean death; grief may mean a procedure not going as planned, the field not being what you hoped it would be, or some other complicated situation that is heart-wrenching. The difficulty of not managing grief as it comes and goes can impact a person's long-term well-being. It often manifests in less obvious ways that do not seem linked, like irritability, disconnection, emotional numbness, and brain fog. Adding more time is one of those things that cannot be changed. However, you can take a moment and a breath to acknowledge that the situation sucked. You can also accept that you are grieving as you feel angry, guilty, sad, or like a zombie on the way home. I wish that more veterinarians valued the need to check in with colleagues who may have experienced a difficult moment and pick up their slack while they process it. The time for grief does not have to be immediately after the incident. It also does not have to be a huge production of emotions. Sometimes, it is just a quick moment to be sad or sometimes to process things on the way home.

In addition to the vulnerabilities listed above, veterinarians also experience a high rate of poor sleep quality and compromised sleep hygiene. This is likely due to a large number of ethical dilemmas racing through your brain, high rates of substance use as a means of avoidance, and limited time at work to rest and process all of this within a culture that does not endorse rest (Ho *et al.*, 2023). The brain needs sleep to work at its full potential and process stress within the day. Poor sleep habits are linked to lower academic performance and lower productivity (Ho *et al.*, 2023). The old "I will sleep when I am dead" saying just doesn't hold up.

In addition to mental stressors in the field, people often struggle with physical pain as well. Being on your feet, lifting animals, bending over in an awkward position to inspect an animal, and other work-related physical stress lead to high levels of physical pain. With little space given to take care of emotional needs, many are likely not stretching, going to physical therapy, or taking care of their physical needs as well. In addition to this, high levels of stress can lead to long periods of time with tightened muscles, hypertension, and other stress-related disorders. Due to the high physical workload, veterinarians often struggle with cardiovascular and musculoskeletal disorders, stress, and fatigue (Hilton, Burke and Signal, 2023). Over time, pain and not being able to achieve at the physical level you once did can be draining and demoralizing. It is also difficult to manage other emotions when a person is in physical pain, as it takes the focus. It's hard to live life to the fullest with chronic pain.

Currently, there is little space for recognizing rewards and accomplishments in day-to-day actions within the field; however, there is ample space for discussing areas for improvement and mistakes (Hilton, Burke and Signal, 2023). We can all do better; however, this does not mean we are not doing things well right now. No wonder you're neurotic, burnt-out, and score low on well-being assessments. I hope that you will be a better veterinarian 5 years from now than you are right now, and even better 5 years after that. This does not mean you are a bad veterinarian; it simply means you can be better. All of the vulnerabilities require a great amount of personal sacrifice. The struggle is not seen or discussed, leading to powerlessness.

There is also a trickle effect to burnout that creates growth in a culture of unhappy people. Unhappy individuals may step into leadership roles, creating a culture of unhappiness that permeates the entire system. When this becomes pervasive in a field, it is difficult to make changes quickly. It becomes expected for people to be burnt-out and struggle as the norm, rather than the exception. People are often perceived as weak for expressing a need for improvement in their well-being. A blind eye is turned to the problem. I am seeing changes, and I am thrilled that the field is discussing well-being more than they have before. There is also a lot of struggle that needs to continue to be addressed.

WHY WAS THERE A SHIFT

Well-being in the veterinary field was not always seen as a problem. Was this because the issue was not discussed, or was there no problem? For many years, veterinarians were primarily seen with livestock and were male. This is a population that did not discuss their struggles. There was a "pick yourself up by your bootstraps" mentality. It is unknown how much stress a veterinarian had during these times, but I can imagine it may have been very different. The growth of companion animals added to the field has added extra layers of expectation and emotion to the job that may not have existed in earlier veterinary work. People are now managing the complex emotions of caregivers who love their pets as family, and contradictory opinions about how someone should treat a companion animal.

In addition to the growth of companion animals, there were some other shifts in the field as well. In just 35 years, the field of veterinary medicine moved from "women are too sensitive and cannot carry out male tasks" to the field being 62% female (Dickson, 2023). There is an increase in expectations when women enter the workforce, especially in a traditionally male-dominated field. Women started the field by having to prove to those around them that they were just as competent as their male counterparts, and they continued to do this. Throughout history and into the present day, women are more likely to be questioned for their decision-making and more likely to receive verbal abuse (Dickson, 2023). Yes, this is infuriating, but there is a reality that while more women are becoming CEO's and high-level business people, women in general are still marginalized in certain situations. Once again, perfectionism and expectations creep in, adding to the pressure of being a female in an authoritative medical role.

Outside of a huge gender switch in the field, veterinary medicine has changed drastically in the last 30 years in other ways as well. There has been a significant shift in technology, which has enhanced animal care. While technological change has allowed the quality and duration of animals' lives to increase, it also increases the expectation from handlers that there will be an answer. Prices also increase as technology advances, creating added pressure for the veterinarian and the handler.

As humans, we like to think we adapt well to change, but every day in my office, I talk to people about the difficulty of change. Knowing what to expect daily is a safe life, good and bad. People can feel unsafe and unsettled when things change, especially when those changes occur quickly. There is sometimes a feeling of not knowing what to expect from your surroundings, which can be difficult. The field of veterinary medicine has been changing swiftly in many different ways. This can be unsettling to all, especially when we don't talk about it.

RETENTION

High stress and low morale lead to low retention. With fewer veterinarians in the field and an increasing number of people drawn to companion animals, the field is struggling to provide the necessary care for the animals in their communities. Schools are making some shifts and creating more programs, some states are adding more lower-level veterinary positions, the conversation is in the wind, but if we don't take care of each other, people will continue to leave the field. This puts additional strain on the veterinary professionals who are currently in the field. In the American Animal Hospital Association's (2024) retention paper, 30% of veterinarians surveyed are planning on leaving the field. They are doing so due to low compensation, a lack of appreciation, and difficulties in continuing their education. The very biased opinion of a mental health therapist speaking; if we cultivate resilience to stress and discuss how to manage the emotions associated with day-to-day tasks while shifting the culture to prioritize caring for one another at all levels, people will be more likely to stay in the field. More veterinarians staying means less strain and better quality within the field.

People often enter the field of veterinary medicine with the expectation that they will be able to apply their values to the work. They expect to be able to set boundaries with their time, money, and decision-making. When working for an agency that does not prioritize well-being, people are given something different from what they expected. Veterinary professionals want to apply their individual knowledge, skills, and belief systems. They want to feel appreciated (American Animal Hospital Association, 2024). Appreciation is complicated in a field that has high rates of neuroticism. People who fit the criteria for neurosis are more likely to see events as problematic (Lecec-Tosevski, Vukovic and Stepaniovic, 2011). With the focus on what can be done better in each procedure and little focus on what was done well, people feel unappreciated for their hard work. People are left feeling trapped and defeated, unable to perform at their best. Low job appreciation directly predicts not just leaving a job role but the whole profession (Hilton, Burke and Signal, 2023). There is a trickle-down effect when the management of clinics presents this way to their staff, leaving all staff feeling like they perform in a less-than-satisfactory way. In the American Animal Hospital Association's (2024) paper, they found that administrators interpreted appreciation as a need for thank you notes, while staff reported feeling appreciated by higher compensation and benefits. There seems to be a disconnect between what appreciation means.

While resilience and all of the topics and skills discussed in this book are widely important in growing retention, there is only so much resilience that one can have in working conditions that do not cater to mental well-being. Change needs to occur at all levels of veterinary medicine for meaningful change to take place. When higher-level personnel in veterinary medicine start prioritizing their mental well-being and resilience, the field will change as a whole. While I repeatedly emphasize in this book that we are working on you as an individual, it is also vital to note that the owners of the practice, practice managers, and higher-ups may also be reading these skills and making positive changes in that aspect of veterinary medicine. I wish people would remember that workplaces can be abusive environments, just like relationships. Advocating for your needs and educating others on the importance of support in your workplace is essential. If your workplace does not fit your needs, it is okay to explore other options.

POSITIVE CHANGE

Unfortunately, when someone is working on change, the focus is often on what is not going well. However, it is just as important to discuss positive changes that have started to happen within the field. People recognize well-being as an important part of keeping veterinarians in the field. There is an increase in culture surrounding mental health and well-being. There has been a call to action with the veterinary school to begin discussing the hardness of the job and how to take care of yourself (Waitz-Kudla *et al.*, 2023). Someone even called on me to write this book, seeing a need for a change in well-being.

I notice people deciding not to leave their careers when they feel that patient-based services are not for them. Instead, people are choosing to focus on coaching and mentoring others to improve their well-being. People crave well-being courses, filling up lecture halls with the hope of building resilience and enjoying their jobs again. Mental health is still stigmatized, but there is a change happening: More people are asking questions and wanting to grow. I see organizations establishing themselves, like NOMV (Not One More Vet) and Mentor Vet, which work toward establishing well-being in the field.

In 2023, when I first spoke at a veterinary conference, I expected a small, select the amount of people sitting in my room discussing well-being. Instead, it was standing room only, and a vast number of people thanking me for the topic. This speaks to how much individuals crave answers for well-being.

I speak to practice owners building practices designed to keep well-being in mind. I watch large franchise companies build facilities not just for the comfort of the animals but for the comfort of the employees as well. The movement toward well-being is happening. Unfortunately, change takes time, especially change that is stigmatized and shunned for many, many years. A significant cultural shift will not happen overnight, but the present growth will build upon itself, and hopefully, in the coming years, the conversations will become larger. Eventually, everything will become natural, and we will not need the conversation at all. My utopian dream is always to work myself out of the job, and I hope the veterinary field builds itself to not need me (or people like me) in the coming years in the same way they need me now.

Not only is the stigma around well-being being broken the stigma around mental health is also starting to be challenged. According to Merks's (2023) white paper, more veterinarians are reaching out for counseling than in any of the previous years. More clinics are offering EAP services (a certain number of free therapy sessions to address a single issue, which is paid for by the clinic).

We need a growing number of colleagues helping each other at all levels and building non-judgmental cultures that treat perfectionism and high expectations of the field, along with lower workloads, healthy interpersonal interactions, and genuine appreciation (da Silva *et al.*, 2023). These shifts are happening, and I hope to see them continue to happen in the years to come.

PERSONALITY PREDISPOSITIONS

It is known that there are personality predispositions that create an increased likelihood that a person will experience burnout in their life. The "five-factor personality trait" test is often given when discussing these predispositions. The personality traits within the model are agreeableness, conscientiousness, extraversion, neuroticism, and openness. Studies have found that agreeableness has a negative correlation with burnout; however, it can also lead to emotional exhaustion. Conscientiousness also has a negative correlation to burnout out however, there is a correlation between conscientiousness and lower work performance as well as emotional exhaustion. Openness also has a negative correlation to burnout, showing an increase in the ability to adapt to change. Extraversion also has a negative correlation to burnout, a potentially related connection to well-being. However, there is a strong correlation to neurosis and burnout across the board (Angelini, 2023). Does that mean that we should all conform to a particular way of being? That is not realistic in the reality of day-to-day living. Instead, learning how to understand your disposition and how it can be a strength allows you to gain resilience in both your strengths and weaknesses.

GIVING UP ON NEUROSIS

This word may be jarring and pejorative to some, but it is used with great intention. The word neurosis is used to describe a personality trait and is cited in many research papers as one of the risk factors within the veterinary field. Oxford Language Dictionary defines Neurosis as: "a mental condition that is not caused by organic disease, involving symptoms of stress (depression, anxiety, obsessive behavior) but not radical loss of touch with reality. 2. excessive and irrational anxiety or obsession." Sadly, it is an offensive word to so many people. It is the aftermath of a mal-nurtured nervous system. It is an extreme of perfectionism that leads to very uncomfortable emotions.

Part of neurosis is also cynicism and negative thinking. Believe it or not, this is a skill we teach people when they are anxious. We discuss coping ahead and knowing how to manage ahead of time so that you know you can tolerate the situation no matter what. The problem becomes when it turns into ruminating thoughts. You feel like you cannot manage the worry thoughts, and they are no longer a coping skill; they now get in the way of the wellness in your life. Neurosis becomes complaining instead of problem-solving. This happens when we get blinders on. Imagine a horse with blinders. They only see ahead of them so as not to be startled by things happening in their peripheral vision. We tend to put emotional blinders on during difficult or high-stress situations. We can only see the negative and difficult parts of life, and the not-so-bad and positive parts of life are left unseen. Our brain develops this initially as a coping mechanism to be prepared for the hard parts of life, but it works too well and the positive becomes dangerous. Your body believes that if you see any of the positives, it will lead to missing something important. This is usually a subconscious coping mechanism and something people do not sign up for. Once you notice that cynicism is showing up in your life, you can start to see thoughts as preparation and use them in the way they are originally designed. We can also begin to challenge ourselves to notice the not-so-bad so that we can start to test the blinders and see the picture, which is usually both positive and negative.

Veterinarians often have a level of perfectionism and want to do things right all of the time. Perfectionism is not always a negative trait; it gets you through veterinary school and improves the quality of your service for the animals. However, it is taken too far when most veterinarians believe they are failing professionally at some level (Dickson, 2023). I have attended conferences and seen firsthand how many people are involved in the world of veterinary medicine. I find it hard to believe that every single person is failing professionally. The reality is that veterinarians care deeply for the animals they are serving; it would be hard to join the profession without that care. With that care comes a desire to give the animal the best treatment possible- striving for perfection because that is what the animal deserves. However, when perfectionism becomes neurosis, it can get in the way of things and make your life pretty hard. You are unlikely to be perfect because flaws happen. When your end goal is perfectionism, this can be defeating and exhausting. It can lead to self-doubt, overthinking, difficulty in stressful situations, and being overwhelmed.

Neurosis is often associated with individuals who are very organized, diligent in their work, and detail-oriented. However, it is also linked to low efficiency and a tendency to have more negative emotions about their work on a more regular basis (da Silva *et al.*, 2023). With every strength comes a weakness and vice versa. It is our job to ensure that both the strengths and weaknesses are evident.

It is not uncommon for veterinarians to show their neurosis when discussing mental well-being skills. I often hear, "Did I do that right?" or "How does this look for me?" or "Can you go over that again so I can get it right?" People tend to want to know all the details to ensure they are perfectly applying each skill. This often leads to not practicing the skill out of fear of doing it incorrectly. I can guarantee that if you do not apply what you learn in this book, it will not be effective. Perfectionism also takes away from curiosity. How can you know if it works if you are concentrating more on your ability to perform the skill than on its effectiveness?

For the sake of this book, I ask that if you struggle with anxiety and neurosis, please set it aside for a moment. It will probably come in and out because it is an integral part of you. Just notice it and set it aside again. You cannot fail in well-being; you can only grow and thrive. Skills not working and concepts not applying are merely knowledge that will help you decide the best way to be. These concepts and skills are not designed to be perfect; they are simply intended to change stuff up slightly so that you have more space for managing things naturally. Trying to do things perfectly can complicate the concepts in the book. If well-being skills create more stress and anxiety, they will exacerbate the problem, not alleviate it. You cannot do them wrong if you are trying them.

Don't worry. If you need to, you can bring your neurosis and perfectionism back for other tasks in your life; please do. It is an essential part of who you are.

Jane is burnt out from working in her job in a large clinic. She feels stuck and is questioning leaving the field altogether. She loves helping animals and feels a deep connection to them, but is unsure if the work is worth it. She reads this book as a last-ditch effort to see if anything will work to bring back the passion she had at the beginning of veterinary school. The concepts seem weird to her, and she does not have much time, but she decides to read a section of a chapter once a week and apply the concepts throughout the day. She is skeptical and wonders if this will just add to her exhaustion. In the first week, she reads the section and decides to try a new routine. The first day, she forgets. She is mad at herself and feels ashamed. "I cannot even do these simple tasks. I am doomed," (her neurosis is talking). Then, she remembers to be kinder to herself when applying these skills. She wakes up the next day and puts her pant leg in a different leg. "This is so weird," she thinks, but she continues. She notices that part of her routine right now is dread, starting with putting on work clothes (She is outside of autopilot, so things feel more accessible). That is interesting, but I did not even notice that. She makes a note to write in her journal about this for 4 minutes when she gets home. She has a glimmer of hope that today might be different. She still dreads work but wonders if it may be better one day. She got in the car and noticed the gas gauge was empty. Dread kicks in again, "Just one more thing in this complicated life." She is super discouraged. "See, I cannot even get better at well-being." She gets gas and gets back in. Something reminds her that it is not supposed to be perfect or instant. She gets to work and remembers the glimmer of hope. This gives a smaller glimmer but something. She is only on day two. She argues with herself, "If this does not work, what will." vs "You are only on day two." She gets home that night and crashes into bed. She wakes up early and remembers not doing the journal she intended to do. "What is wrong with me? I cannot follow through with anything." She decides to journal about this. She is very harsh to herself in her journal. The timer goes off, and she switches hands. For some reason, this hand makes more sense. "Of course, I forgot I am burnt out and tired. One step at a time, Jane," she thinks. She puts on her pants for work, the other leg this time. She feels the dread, but it doesn't feel as overwhelming today.

Fast forward to a few weeks in. She reads the book on and off and sometimes tries the skills when she can. Some stuff works, and some does not. She is seeing small changes in her life. She wishes it moved faster but has giving herself time to settle into the new concepts. She is still unsure if she wants to stay in the profession, but she can provide space for good moments in her day—the animals she can make a difference with and the handlers who love their pets. The space is small but there. She notices thoughts about "this being weird and dumb" or "It did not work, am I doing it right." She also notices that sometimes she gets frustrated that the process is slow, but she still sees if it might work. Some days, she is pessimistic about the process; others, she has small amounts of hope; some days glimmers of both.

Eventually, Jane notices that she is accidentally regulating her nervous system. She is developing a new autopilot, a new groove that is much healthier. People start responding to her better when she is less frantic and stressed. There is light at the end of the burnout tunnel. Jane messes up a lot in this story. She is even hard on herself. However, the more she notices the neurosis, the more she is able to manage it and apply the skills anyway.

HIGH ACHIEVERS

The idea of high achievers has historically been discussed when talking about successful athletes. In high-level competitive sports, there is a need for large goals and a determination to meet them. High achievement is characterized by a high level of competitiveness, and many high achievers benefit from feeling in control of their environment, which allows them to persevere in difficult situations. However, this poses a risk when external forces are outside of their power, which can be anxiety-producing. Examples of external factors could be expectations from the field, the program, the handlers, or others. Veterinary medicine programs typically accept people who are high academic achievers in their previous education. Veterinary school is rigorous, and these are the people who are more likely to succeed. Because their peers are at a similar level of performance, students may show a level of impostor syndrome as they compare themselves to people around them (Stelling, Mastenbroek and Kremer, 2019). Performance athletes score higher on the scale of conscientiousness, showing strong will, motivation, dutifulness, and commitment, as well as being well organized. It can be seen how this can benefit people as they progress through veterinary school and beyond. This person prefers clearly defined objectives and will work hard to achieve them. While athletes who are practicing in their sport show low rates of neurosis, athletes who are no longer practicing show high rates of neurosis. This makes me wonder if there is something that can be added to the field of veterinary medicine that will allow people to "practice in their sport." Maybe if we change our way of thinking to noticing achievement, we can create the same environment as a high-level sport.

While objectives are wildly obvious in school (get the grade, pass the class, graduate), they are often less defined once someone gets into a career. This can lead them to feel stuck. Perhaps creating objectives for the day, week, or month would be a way to insert the "sport" into the field once again.

RESPONSIBILITY FOR OTHERS' EMOTIONS

It can be very easy to carry the emotional burden of those around us. We become scared that people are mad, feel like we are responsible for making them happy, and have a desire to fix their anxiety. Because we are pack animals, we read the emotions of those around us to establish a sense of community and determine what is safe for ourselves. Alongside the natural tendencies for us to share emotions at a biological level, you care about your job, so you also share emotions related to it. We feel sad with those who feel sad. We feel the joy of the animal being goofy that day. Sometimes you even hold the handler's emotions so much that they become your own.

People coming into a veterinary office are often stressed with the burden of caring for a dearly beloved critter. When a person is under stress, they rarely keep it to themselves. They vent to others, become angry, struggle with decisions, and present very anxious to those around them. Veterinarians are holding these emotions throughout the day for many people. You are the one sitting with the stress of the handler while they wonder if their pet will be okay. When people become anxious, they may talk excessively, ask numerous questions, or present themselves frantically. They may become irritable as they desperately search for answers. They may break down and cry due to overwhelm. This is called a burden transfer. The burden becomes yours as well due to the person's response to emotions. This is a lot of energy to hold when you are simply trying to help an animal (Laura *et al.*, 2024).

The reason people present so outwardly is because they want a fix to their struggle. The problem is there is not always a fix, but your body system will likely match their desire for a fix, creating a level of frantic for yourself. You, too, will find yourself wanting to fix the stress-causing situation for their comfort, but also for your own. Our system wants to keep us comfortable, which means keeping the other person comfortable.

You are sitting with sadness as people find out that their pet is sicker than they hoped, or their bill is too much for them to afford. As humans, we typically do not want people to be sad. We share the grief thinking of animals we have felt attached to that we lost, and the despair that can sometimes come with grief. We sometimes feel very connected to the animal, and we grieve their death ourselves.

High rates of burnout and large amounts of burden transfer are directly correlated (Laura *et al.*, 2024). This, along with a need to be seen and appreciated, may be the most significant vulnerabilities within the field. This is not something we can make go away. Some of the emotions we need to hold for other people to do well at our job. The struggle becomes when it is difficult to tell what we need to work with and empathize with, and what we need to let go of because we have no control over the situation, no matter how much the handler wants us to.

In addition to burden transfer, the job tells you to have good customer service. When I talk to veterinarians, they interpret this differently than in some other fields. There is a fear that people will become angry, write an online review, and the clinic will never recover. People are willing to accept abuse, sway on policy, and do what it takes to make the customer happy. It's interesting because not even Costco offers that kind of customer service, and they will even take back your Christmas tree after Christmas. Within this need for customer service, veterinarians respond in a way that frantically needs to please the customers, sometimes holding the comfort of the client above the needs of the staff.

FOOD FOR THOUGHT JOURNALING:

1. What gets in the way of your well-being success?

2. How can this barrier also be a strength?

REFERENCES

Angelini, G. (2023). 'Big five model personality traits and job burnout: a systematic literature review', *BMC Psychology*, 11(1), p. 49.

American Animal Hospital Association (2018) *AAHA's guide to veterinary practice team wellbeing* [White paper]. Available at: https://www.aaha.org/wp-content/uploads/globalassets/04-practice-resources/practice-culture/team_wellbeing_guide.pdf

American Animal Hospital Association (2024) *Stay, please: Veterinary medicine has a problem—it's losing good people at an unsustainable rate.* Available at: https://www.aaha.org

Cooney, K. and Kipperman, B. (2023). 'Ethical and practical considerations associated with companion animal euthanasia', *Animals*, 13(3), 430. https://doi.org/10.3390/ani13030430.

da Silva, C. R. *et al.* (2023). 'Suicide in veterinary medicine: A literature review', *Veterinary World*, 16(6), pp. 1266–1276. https://doi.org/10.14202/vetworld.2023.1266-1276.

Dickson, B. (2023) *Ethical dilemmas and moral distress in companion animal veterinary medicine: Mental health implications.* Unpublished manuscript. https://scholars.wlu.ca/cgi/viewcontent.cgi?article=3771&context=etd.

Hilton, K. R., Burke, K. J. and Signal, T. (2023). 'Mental health in the veterinary profession: An individual or organisational focus?', *Australian Veterinary Journal*, 101(1–2), pp. 41–48 https://doi.org/10.1111/avj.13215.

Ho, N. T., Santoro, F., Palacios Jimenez, C. and Pelligand, L. (2023). 'Cross-sectional survey of sleep, fatigue and mental health in veterinary anaesthesia personnel', *Veterinary Anaesthesia and Analgesia*, 50(4), pp. 315–324. https://doi.org/10.1016/j.vaa.2023.03.003.

Laura, L., Arapović, M., Duvnjak, S. and Arapović, J. (2024). 'Empathy and mental health in veterinary medicine', *Veterinary Research Communications*, 48(4), pp. 1991–1997.

Lecec-Tosevski, D., Vukovic, O. and Stepaniovic, J. (2011). 'Stress and personality', *Psychiatriki*, 22(4), pp. 290–297.

Merks, J. (2023). 'Veterinary wellbeing study', *Journal of Veterinary Science*, pp. 1–15.

Smith, E. T., Barcelos, A. M. and Mills, D. S. (2023). 'Links between pet ownership and exercise on the mental health of veterinary professionals', *Veterinary Record Open*, 10(1), e62. https://doi.org/10.1002/vro2.62.

Smits, F. (2022) *Autistic veterinary surgeons in the United Kingdom: Workplace stressors and mental wellbeing* [Master of Research Thesis, University of Nottingham]. Available at: http://eprints.nottingham.ac.uk/78517/1/14324658_Femke%20Smits_MRES%20thesis%20corrections.pdf

Stelling, A. G., Mastenbroek, N. J. and Kremer, W. D. (2019). 'Predictive value of three different selection methods for admission of motivated and well-performing veterinary medical students', *Journal of Veterinary Medical Education*, 46(3), pp. 289–301.

Waitz-Kudla, S. N., Kramper, S., Roark, A., Mani, I. and Witte, T. K. (2023). 'Securing lethal means for suicide: A focus group study exploring perceptions and barriers among practicing veterinarians', *Journal of the American Veterinary Medical Association*, 261(11), pp. 1683–1693.

Mental Well-Being in the Veterinary Field

People outside the field do not often see the struggles that veterinarians face. The stress and overwhelm are usually hidden by customer service and misconceptions. It is challenging to share the difficult aspects of the job with family and friends, and it is unprofessional to share the struggles with handlers. In addition, they may sometimes feel unseen by the animals. While the logical brain reminds us that the animals do not feel safe around us because they do not understand we are there to help, and they are scared, we can sometimes take it personally when they snap or try to protect themselves. Handlers, family, and friends sometimes snap in a similar way, but it's even harder to understand their natural instincts. Veterinarians have hidden their struggle for many years, powering through without anyone knowing what it looks like behind the mask. There is shame in talking to friends who are veterinarians, after all, we all chose the job and should be able to manage our emotions within it. There is a misunderstood feeling when talking to nonveterinary friends. They love hanging out with animals, so it must be fun to be a vet, plus their bills are high, so you must get paid well. This leads to a sense of being stuck and veterinarians feeling like they have to figure it out on their own. An impossible task when things get the hardest.

I am not a veterinarian, and I have a pet dog, which makes me *gasp* at the general public. When I talk to friends, colleagues, and random people I play golf with about my work with veterinarians, they are often confused. It is not uncommon to have a conversation that goes something like this:

ME: "I have been working with veterinarians to build their resilience and well-being lately."

THEM: "Veterinarians (in a shocked voice)"

ME: "Yes, they are really struggling. They have high mental health rates and the highest rates of suicide than any other profession."

THEM: "Really? Veterinarians?"

ME: "Yes, They have a very stressful job. Think about it: everyone coming into their office is worried about their animal; they know they will have a high bill and are grouchy. Veterinarians get mistreated a lot."

THEM: "I guess that makes sense."

ME: "In addition, they are a low-paid profession."

THEM: "Really? My veterinary bills are high."

ME: "Yes, but veterinary medicine has many expenses. They keep an inventory of meds; they have to pay for space and all the equipment that comes with it and have high student loan payments. It's not all about the face-to-face."

THEM: "I guess I never thought about that."

ME: "They are also faced with a lot of emotions. They have to make decisions for people's animals daily, and sometimes that decision means encouraging euthanasia."

THEM: "Oh wow."

ME: "Plus, they went into the field to work with animals, but they must deal with us."

THEM: "Good point."

Outside of the people you know, love, and complain to, people do not understand the struggle. Sometimes your loved ones don't quite understand it either. You have all the stress of human medicine with less recognition. Don't be afraid to tell people about the struggles in your profession (at the right time, of course, don't just complain everywhere you look). The only way to gain awareness is to educate people around you. I will be doing the same.

Other healthcare professionals tend to get entirely different responses. Human counterparts are thanked for their hard work and acknowledged for the challenges their job presents. When I say I am working with a nurse or a doctor or even another therapist, people understand that they must feel exhausted, burnt-out, and struggling. I don't know why this is different, but maybe it is because veterinarians zip it up a bit better, stay in the background, and are silent about the hard work of the job.

Stress is not isolated to the job that you work. You are still living life as you are working. When you are already stressed with day-to-day struggles outside of work, you will be more susceptible to the day-to-day stress of work life (Lecec-Tosevski, Vukovic and Stepaniovic, 2011).

Traditionally, when a large group of people is struggling with low well-being scores, professionals attribute the struggle to difficult childhoods. It is assumed that due to a stressful early life, it is harder to manage life today. While our past does impact our ability to cope, it is not the only reason people may struggle. Researchers call the struggles that people may have in their childhood adverse childhood experiences (ACEs). They include childhood trauma, low income, living with someone with mental health or substance abuse, bullying, incarceration, and natural disasters. While these would affect a person's well-being, veterinary medicine has not shown a significant difference in ACE scores compared to the general public (Strand *et al.*, 2017). With mental health scores higher, well-being scores lower, and ACE studies the same, what makes veterinary medicine struggle?

American Animal Hospital Association's research (2018) states that veterinarians want to be valued. This is true for any job or really human. We all need a purpose and must understand how it contributes to the community. For veterinarians, this is especially important because, as I speak with people in the veterinary field, many identify that a large part of their identity often lies in their work. Many factors contribute to the difficulty in feeling valued, and there are many pieces alongside the need to be valued; however, being seen and valued is a core struggle within the field.

BURNOUT, COMPASSION FATIGUE, AND VICARIOUS TRAUMA

You may have heard the common words referring to struggles in the workplace: burnout, compassion fatigue, and vicarious trauma. These words describe our long-term reaction to an untreated stressful work environment. All healthcare professionals and responders suffer from these work-related stressors; they are not isolated to veterinary professionals. However, they present differently within each profession due to the specific stressors within the field. While burnout, compassion fatigue, and vicarious trauma often overlap, some nuances create some differences between each.

BURNOUT

I feel confident you have heard people talk of burnout at some point in your life. The topic is increasing in popularity. Sometimes it is correct content, sometimes it is exaggerated. Burnout is more than just not liking your job, your boss, your company, or being mad at handlers. Sometimes we do not like our job or parts of our job. Sometimes we do not like working and wish we could magically become independently wealthy. This is not burnout. Burnout goes deeper than this; it presents as a persistent feeling of being stuck that we can't shake. It often haunts us both on the job and off the job. It also doesn't happen overnight; there is usually a progression of symptoms that eventually lead to burnout.

Sometimes we notice these symptoms while we are living in them; other times they sneak up on us, and it feels like we wake up one day, unhappy with everything. We may start wondering where our place is in our careers. We begin to disconnect from those around us, still doing our job and enjoying it, but not feeling connected. We feel less motivated to do the parts of our job we like a little less. We are not quite burnt-out, but we are inching that way. I have heard this middle ground informally called "brown out." People often push the first symptoms under the rug. People expect them as they know they work in a stressful career. People believe that "this is the way it should be." They do not talk about it because they think people around them are doing a better job of managing the stress than they are (I can tell you as a therapist who sees the deep dark secrets of the general public, most aren't). They feel ashamed and fear people will say they are not coping well. They know what they need to do (exercise, eat healthy, meditate), but they just can't do it. All the shame makes people feel like they need to hide their struggle as deeply as possible. They pick themselves up, put on their big girl panties, and put on a face of happiness. Not sharing struggles with others not only creates isolation and loneliness, but it also creates additional shame around a secret. We communicate that we must be doing something wrong if we aren't sharing it. Now we not only have burnout symptoms, but we also have shame around the burnout symptoms. In addition, emotions can never be completely hidden and eventually turn into deep, painful burnout. When a person is burnt-out, they feel so disconnected from work, feeling that it has no meaning. This is especially difficult in passion-driven careers like veterinary medicine.

Burnout, by definition, has three key characteristics: emotional exhaustion, a sense of disconnection from oneself and one's job, and lower performance. Many also add cognitive and emotional distress to this definition. These symptoms may look similar to depression, and, untreated, it can become diagnosable depression; however, unlike depression, burnout speaks specifically to the job as opposed to a generalization to one's entire life. Some people discuss the two as one and define burnout as work-related depression (Schaufeli *et al.*, 2023; Schaufeli, Desart and De Witte, 2020). It is unlikely for people to use these exact words when they are describing burnout. Below is a list of words and symptoms you may hear or see when you or someone you know is burnt-out. If many of these feel familiar, you may be experiencing burnout.

Emotionally exhausted	Avoiding work	Feeling a desire to avoid people associated with work	Fanticizing about no longer having a job	No longer connecting with patients	Feeling annoyed by things you used to feel empathy toward
Feeling irritable much of the time	Never feeling rested on workdays	Not feeling any emotions during the day	Feeling like your emotions take over, and you have no control	Parts of your job you used to like now feels like chores	Making more mistakes
Brain Fog	Feeling outside your body (feeling like you are looking at yourself doing tasks)	Only noticing stress and yuck of the day while struggling to see successes	Feeling deep shame for small mistakes	Having a hard time remembering information	Feeling like you are going through the motions of the job without any connection
Calling out sick more	Physically moving more slowly in the clinic	Increasing substance use to avoid thoughts	Ruminating thoughts about not liking your job	Obsessively complaining about parts of the job	Feeling stuck and unable to leave
Nihilism	Loss of direction	Feeling adrift			

Burnout is found in all helping professions, but is exceptionally prevalent among veterinarians. Well-being study reports that 74% of veterinarians experience medium to high burnout levels. When rates are this high, it becomes a norm and an expectation in the field (Manning *et al.*, 2024). People often expect to be miserable because of the field they have chosen to pursue. It becomes whiny to discuss it and impossible for changes to be made. It can even become contagious, like lobsters in a bucket of burnout, pulling each other in. Many times, people feel like leaving the field is the only way they can survive the feelings of burnout. I notice people moving to less client-centered jobs to avoid the lifestyle that leads to burnout. With a shortage of veterinarians, this is really scary for an already struggling profession.

Good news. There are ways to treat burnout without having to change careers. When we regulate our nervous system in relation to our job using the concepts and skills in this book, we can realign with our authentic selves, which naturally helps us avoid burnout and enables effective decision-making regarding our career.

Example *Genevieve has been working in veterinary medicine for 3 years. She has been working at a large clinic that treats many animals daily. Her boss is very financially focused and disconnected from the workers around her. The handlers expect immediate answers to all of their questions and are very demanding. She used to love the small animals she worked with. She has a few people at work she smiles and makes small talk with, but does not feel connected to any of the other workers. Everyone is pretty grouchy in the clinic. She once mentioned to her direct boss that she thinks the handlers do not respect veterinarians, and she was told, "This is part of the job." She cognitively knows that she is good at her job, but she often discredits her knowledge, making her take longer on each case. Her boss has noticed this and tells her she needs to speed up the work. Lately, when she comes to work, she feels like she disconnects from her entire self and goes through the motions of work. She is not connecting to the animals like she once did and rarely makes eye contact with the handler. She has been making small mistakes, which her boss has also pointed out. She worries the mistakes will get bigger, so she tries harder, but it feels impossible. The more she tries to be more detail-oriented, the more mistakes she seems to make. She often gets in the car after work and wants to cry, but doesn't seem able to. She is so tired from disconnecting throughout the day that she goes home, watches trash television, and goes to bed. When her friends reach out, she avoids their desire to hang out, feeling as though she doesn't have the time. She used to enjoy working out before work, but she has let this slide to have a more comfortable time in bed. Every day, she hopes that there is some reason that the clinic will be closed and daydreams about disasters that create a day off. She is ashamed of these thoughts as they seem pretty grim. She feels very stuck and wonders if she chose the right career, but having wanted to be a veterinarian her entire life, she is unsure where else to turn. She has contemplated changing jobs, but she worries it will be the same everywhere she goes, and is worried she is not good enough at her job. Genevieve is burnt out.*

COMPASSION FATIGUE

Compassion Fatigue is the inability to feel compassionate emotions toward patients. It presents itself with poor bedside manner, difficulty listening, and difficulty empathizing with the patient. You can show compassion fatigue for the animal, the handler, or both. The job becomes cold and heartless, and people in this space often just show up and go through the motions. Compassion fatigue usually comes from caring for patients in a way that we embody the feelings and feel like we are living the struggle of the patient as if it is our own. I have heard this referred to as holding empathy (feeling the feelings as if they are your own) versus compassion (feeling sad for a person while also knowing it is not yours). Burden transfer refers to the idea that we hold the emotions of others around us. Young veterinarians tend to hold this burden until it becomes too much, and then transition to compassion fatigue. It can be challenging to find a balance where we show empathy for our handlers and animals while also not taking on their burden.

Compassion fatigue not only comes from holding the burden of those around us, but it can also come when we avoid the very real emotions of the job and shove them down, not returning to them to allow them to complete themselves. The nervous system begins to define compassion and all other emotions we feel in the day-to-day work of the job as a dangerous response. When we have not managed these emotions effectively and avoid them, they are no longer safe to feel, even if we need them. Unfortunately, when we avoid and turn off an emotion, we cannot pick and choose which emotions we feel. They all become unavailable, and compassion fatigue sets in.

Sometimes, compassion fatigue is very conscious, and you can see it very clearly; sometimes, it is more subconscious and takes others to point it out to you. Compassion fatigue may sound glorious to those who have empathized deeply with others around them. Empathy can feel painful at times. However, it is often difficult to contain compassion fatigue to just work, leading to an impact on personal relationships. It can sometimes lead to feelings of guilt that you no longer care, disconnection from everyone in your life, and irritability toward anyone who shows emotion.

I often hear that an emotional disconnect is necessary for high-stress jobs that involve large emotions. Compassion fatigue is praised as an effective coping mechanism. I understand where this construct comes from; however, it is not true. The reality is that full emotional disconnect makes people less effective at their jobs. It can be easier to miss small details that may be important in prognosis. You may also lose clients because they see you as cold and difficult to connect to. Moreover, over time, it also leads to a mistrust of the entire field from those receiving services. Instead of emotionally disconnecting, I encourage people to recognize that emotions are high, work toward logical compassion for the other people in the room, and eventually look introspectively, allowing time for the high emotions to process. Our perception in the moment tells us that it is easier to ignore the emotions and disconnect. However, emotions do not do well-being ignored, and eventually this disconnection leads to problematic behavior. Trust me, I see the tail end of it when it no longer works. I acknowledge that at a surface level, it feels easier just to power through, but I can assure you, compassion fatigue is exhausting in its own way.

As with many parts of life, there is a middle ground. We cannot feel all the emotions all the time, especially when we are working on multiple cases back-to-back throughout the entire day. It is necessary to set aside a difficult case while you work with the next patient. The struggle arises when you fail to check in on yourself at the end of the day. Believe it or not, our body holds a natural release valve when we listen to it. It will allow us to feel our emotions in bursts instead of title waves. The unfortunate part is that it works best once our emotions are perceived by our nervous system as safe, which means we can feel them without being overwhelmed by them.

Example *Mira works in an emergency veterinary clinic and has for 5 years. When she started in the clinic she would often spend large amounts of time with the handlers. She would provide grief resources when needed and allow space for them to cry in a room before they left, especially when they felt overwhelmed. She used to leave exhausted from all the emotions. Lately, she notices that every person who comes in is "just one more case." She goes through the motions of providing care for each patient, but becomes increasingly annoyed when someone begins to grieve or feel anxious about their pet. She often thinks, "You and everyone else." When pets are agitated due to their distress, she becomes very annoyed, wondering, "I am trying to help you, ugh." When she treats an animal and things go well, she moves on to the next case. Never leaving time for her accomplishments. In the back room, she talks with her co-workers about how annoying everyone is who comes in. Mira is experiencing Compassion fatigue.*

VICARIOUS TRAUMA/SECONDARY TRAUMA

While I have heard vicarious trauma and secondary trauma used interchangeably, there is a small distinction between the two. Vicarious Trauma speaks to a gradual development of trauma responses related to prolonged exposure to stressful experiences. Secondary trauma speaks to feeling trauma as if it is you when treating an animal or a person who has experienced a trauma and is related to a single case.

Secondary trauma can be due to several different reasons. Maybe a mistake was made in the procedure, or you feel responsible for the distress of others. Maybe that case reminded us of our own story. Sometimes, this is an obvious connection, such as an animal that reminds us of our own pet, or a person who reminds us of ourselves, or a loved one. Other times it is more hidden. It may be a dynamic of control that hits a nerve or someone with similar traits to someone else in our lives. Sometimes, the stress of a procedure or event can remind us of something we haven't thought of in many years. Something that we did not believe still impacts us. Sometimes we don't know why a certain procedure creates symptoms of secondary trauma; it just does. When someone is experiencing secondary trauma, they often exhibit similar symptoms of Post-Traumatic Stress Disorder. Symptoms of both secondary and vicarious trauma are identical. Vicarious trauma typically presents slowly over time, over the course of several months, while secondary trauma tends to have a more sudden onset. Symptoms of both include:

- Images of the incident when we close our eyes or fall asleep

- Struggling not to think about it due to ruminating thoughts

- Hypervigilance (constantly scanning for danger)

- Jumpiness

- Developing a distorted belief system about yourself or the world

- Feeling like everything is doomed

- Nightmares or sleep disturbance

- Isolation for others

- Avoidance of places or things that will remind you of the situation

- Feeling like you are back in the event, and it is happening again

- Feelings of anxiety or depression (Leris and Byrne, 2003)

It is very easy to chalk these symptoms up to burnout, as they can appear similar; however, they are likely linked to specific types of procedures, animals, or events more than to the entire job. You may notice yourself feeling especially disgusted by something specific in your job, or dreaming about something specific. You notice a trend in the cases that trigger you the most.

When people experience secondary or vicarious trauma, they often develop a negative view of the world. They may feel a general sense of unsafety in their world, struggle to trust others, or have ruminating thoughts that are difficult to manage. They may feel doom about the people and the world in which they live. While we are unsure why some traumatic events are traumatizing and some are not, it is clear that our bodies sometimes do not process difficult situations in the way that they are designed. Based on my studies, I have developed a theory that our body has learned that our beliefs about the events, emotions around the events, or some aspect of the event have been communicated as unsafe to the body. This creates layers that interfere with the natural processing our body needs to overcome critical incident stress.

Unfortunately, it is impossible to avoid all cases that have potential for secondary or vicarious trauma. In fact, to complicate things, avoidance of triggers actually establishes more triggers, making it difficult to treat. Instead of avoiding, we can build skills that foster resilience, making us less likely to be impacted. Skills in this book can create the necessary skills that build safety in the nervous system. This can allow for more space to process stressful events naturally. We can also notice when we are impacted and have a plan for how we will address a struggle. Plan for who you will reach out to (through the shame that makes it difficult to talk about) and what activities you will continue, no matter how hard they may be. Noticing and labeling our struggle without judgment is a first step in managing it.

We do not get to pick when our body starts struggling with vicarious trauma. It is a subconscious reaction. While we know that past trauma and other psychological stressors can be risk factors for vicarious trauma and secondary trauma, we also know that these trauma responses can hit anyone and often do not make logical sense. People tend not to speak of vicarious trauma because they believe it makes them weak, worse at their job, or crazy; however, it is extremely prevalent and very treatable when people are open and honest. I often hear a belief that people are coping worse than people around them due to the symptoms. People often seem unaware that many veterinarians face similar struggles and will experience some form of vicarious or secondary trauma at some point in their career.

While stressful events sometimes become a difficult memory and nothing else, they do not always process naturally. They can become stuck in some form of processing, causing the symptoms to persist for months or years, and can be very uncomfortable for the person experiencing them. I encourage you to seek professional help if you struggle to find relief from your vicarious or secondary trauma symptoms. Many trauma-based therapies are very effective in the treatment of these traumas.

VICARIOUS TRAUMA

Example   *Jason has been working in a high-stress clinic with limited support. He recently had a case where a young puppy was put under anesthesia for a routine dental procedure and passed away during the procedure. While there is always a risk in this procedure, it is unclear what happened that led to the death of the patient. Jason has been replaying the event constantly. When he closes his eyes, he sees the moment they realized the puppy was not responsive. He obsessively tries to find the error that caused the death. He has intrusive memories of the owner's face when they communicated the loss. He has been struggling to perform any tasks effectively at work. He feels constant fear of making more mistakes. He feels that if he talks to his nonveterinary friends about this, they will not understand and will worry about their own pets' well-being during procedures. He worries that if he talks to his veterinary friends about this, they will judge his ability in the field or his ability to manage the stress of the difficult case. He has become reclusive, not talking to anyone. He knows that people often speak about mistakes happening, and the message about being kinder to himself has been all around him, but they don't seem true in this moment. He is struggling to sleep and forces himself to eat one small meal a day. He feels stuck in this case without any way out. Jason is experiencing Secondary Trauma.*

SECONDARY TRAUMA

Example   *Olivia has become very anxious in her day-to-day life. She notices that she is constantly worried that her dog will die when she leaves. As she turns the corner to get to her house after work, she notices that she is holding her breath, worried that her house has burned down with her dog in it, or that she will show up and he will have passed. The thoughts haunt her intermittently throughout the day. She started losing sleep because the worry had sunk into her dreams, waking her in the middle of the night. She has been startlingly easy as well. Just the other day, her vet tech called out her name to* *get her attention about a medication, which made her jump so high that it took some time for her heart rate to return to normal. Olivia is not sure how this all started, but she is beginning to feel crazy. She notices herself avoiding dogs who remind her of her own. Oliva is experiencing vicarious trauma.*

MORAL INJURY AND DECISION-MAKING FATIGUE

Moral injury is also a stress response common in the field of veterinary medicine. Moral injury is when a person feels like a bad person due to an action in their past, many times not see the whole picture outside of personal responsibility. Moral injury is the physiological and psychological response to being a part of something that contradicts your value system. This can be due to a difference of opinion with the animal handler, the agency, or close working colleagues. Moral injury can also arise from making a decision based on your values, but it has an unfortunate outcome, which prompts you to question your morals and values. Moral injury can lead to feeling like a bad person or a cognitive failure, ultimately resulting in a lack of trust in oneself. People sometimes think they do not deserve to feel better, and their symptoms are a punishment for their past.

Moral injury can be found in many professions; however, it may manifest differently in veterinary medicine due to factors specific to the field. Unlike most of the human treating counterparts, in veterinary medicine, the being that is getting treatment is not the one giving consent (Stetina and Krouzecky, 2022). This means that veterinarians may suggest a treatment they believe is best for the animal, and the handler (the one giving consent) does not agree to the treatment being recommended. This can lead to significant discomfort for the patient being treated, who is unable to express their needs. Given that the average veterinarian is presented with upwards of five dilemmas a day (Stetina and Krouzecky, 2022) (either due to conflict with handlers, complex cases, or differences of opinions within the field), it is likely that moral stress will present itself often within the day-to-day life of your career.

Left untreated, this moral stress can lead to moral injury. Physiologically, Moral Injury leads to deep shame and can present itself with responses similar to those of other traumas. (Stetina and Krouzecky, 2022) People often have ruminating thoughts about being a bad person, unlovable, or something similar. This deep feeling of shame can manifest into irritability or a lack of trust in yourself. This lack of trust in yourself leads to decision-making fatigue or moral fatigue (feeling a disconnect from morals and values in decision-making) and burnout, related explicitly to tricky situations and decision-making. This lack of trust in yourself can make it challenging to make the necessary decisions for treatment, ultimately reducing your effectiveness at work.

Moral Injury is often less apparent than its counterparts in the world of work-related stress. It creeps into people's responses slowly, and it is talked about far less. Many times, when treating moral injury in my office, it takes a few sessions to label it for what it is, and even longer for people to admit that it may be related to their work. Left untreated, there is often a gaping hole within a person's intrapersonal self.

Sometimes we do not make it quite to the shame that comes from moral injury, but we do suffer from decision-making fatigue. There comes a time when people become exhausted from making decisions. There are so many major decisions in the day-to-day life of a veterinarian that, likely, some will not turn out the way you wish. You may want to make a different decision or miss a detail. You may begin to question your own decision-making abilities. It becomes challenging to decide where to eat when your family asks; nonetheless, the plan of action for a complicated case. In the case of the hamburger, it is easy to default to those around you. When it comes to the case, it can cause extreme distress in the animal and the staff around you. When decision-making takes longer, it can be really difficult in the fast-paced environment of the clinic.

DECISION FATIGUE

Example *Steph has been working for a veterinarian for 3 years. She learned growing up that you always listen to your superior, and a value of the clinic she works for is that the customer comes first. She is constantly making decisions about the animal's health, and the handlers either follow her advice or don't. Lately, her decisions have taken much longer. She feels frozen periodically throughout the day. When her friends ask her where she would like to grab dinner, her mind goes blank, which is frustrating to them. Her thinking is slower, and her vet techs are becoming frustrated. She wavers back and forth before making a decision and is never quite sure if it is the right one. Even when things go well in the clinic, she ruminates about her decisions, wondering if they were best for the animal, the handler, herself and the clinic.*

MORAL INJURY

Example *Tammy was up late at a concert last night and came into work tired from the night before. This was her favorite band and she didn't want to miss it. She figured she could tolerate one day of being tired. Tammy was working on an animal on a routine procedure, and the dog had a reaction to the anesthesia and passed way. Tammy feels as though the death is her fault and feels like her lack of sleep from the night before played a part in the death. No matter how much she fact checks, and no matter how much other people tell her it is not her fault, she cannot shake the shame. She has started to wonder if she is a bad person and has a desire to isolate in a way that she feels she is protecting others from her flaws. She feels like her friends only ask her to hang out because they feel sorry for her. She struggles to feel connected to herself in the world, often feeling like she is floating around in life. She is unsure where she fits in because she does not feel adequate as a veterinarian, but she also does not feel adequate anywhere else in life. She does not talk to anyone about this, as it seems too complicated and too dark to talk to peers, and she worries she will not be able to articulate her struggles to a therapist. Steph is suffering from moral injury.*

You may notice that many of the work-related stress categories overlap. They tend to intertwine themselves into a knot. You may notice that you identify with parts of all but not all of all. This is not an all-or-nothing topic, which can be difficult for some to digest. You do not have to have all symptoms to meet the criteria for a work-related stress problem. You also do not have to label your distress under one of these categories. While the field of veterinary medicine has natural factors which contribute to these types of distress, and it is likely you will feel some level of some or all work-related stress categories, it is also likely that with awareness and skills, you can feel these symptoms temporarily and can build resilience to feel them less often and for shorter periods of time when they do come up.

LONELINESS

Which came first, the chicken or the egg, loneliness or poor well-being scores? It is hard to tell what came first, as they seem to feed off of each other. Loneliness can come from a myriad of different things. Feeling isolated by communities, a lack of relationship with an intimate person, feeling isolated due to an ailment that makes it hard to socialize, and an internal isolation that can come from secrets, shame, difficulty coping, or low self-esteem (Nashwan *et al.*, 2024). To complicate the treatment of loneliness, when a person feels lonely, they also perceive a lack of support from managers, friends, and family (Kulari and Pereira de Castro, 2024). Because it is unclear whether the perception matches the reality, additional support is often needed in the face of loneliness. This is particularly challenging in the field of veterinary medicine because higher-level employers usually have time constraints and limited emotional capacity to provide the support that is needed when a person is struggling.

As mentioned before, veterinarians tend to internalize struggles related to the field. People outside of the field do not understand their struggle, and people in the field do not have time to listen or may judge you. This internalization can make someone feel like they are different than everyone else and unable to fit in, leading to a high level of loneliness. It also creates shame within the struggle. In addition, the job often expects long and sometimes unpredictable work hours. This can make it challenging to establish new relationships and maintain the ones you already have. A large part of the job incorporates a sharing of space with a high intensity of emotions. The clinic not only has emotionally shared space from those working there, but also the animals under stress and their handlers. Many times, people can feel like they used their energy on these people and have less energy for other people outside of work. With all of the complicated layers within the field, it makes sense that veterinarians and other veterinary professionals would struggle with loneliness.

For those who tend to gain energy from isolated and quiet time, it may feel confusing to feel lonely when they crave the isolation. Loneliness is not necessarily just the difficulty of having human interaction. It is a felt sense that can be real or perceived, which feels as though one is alone in a difficult situation. It does not imply that all people need connection at all times; however, we are pack animals who need some quality social interaction. We all want to be seen and understood. It does not feel good for anyone to feel like they cannot connect with others. Even if you do not gain energy from social interactions, you still need the support of others.

There are many theories about why humans feel sensations of loneliness. Some say the feeling of loneliness is designed to motivate us to connect and support each other. Some theorize that loneliness is based on a lack of connection with our parents, leading to a difficult time connecting for the rest of our lives. Some say it is a logical mismatch between a need to connect and the availability of quality connections. Still others view loneliness as a positive emotion communicating a need for internal growth (Nashwan *et al.*, 2024). In my opinion, all of these theories can co-exist at once. Yes, loneliness has the intention of motivating us to connect. Still, when it is intense and outside of our emotional window, it actually creates a level of disconnection from each other, exacerbating the feeling. A person growing up with a family that is emotionally disconnected may not learn how to connect in a way that allows them to thrive in adult life; however, this does not mean these feelings cannot be healed or repaired. Loneliness can be a positive sensation, encouraging more growth, but this can only be part of the struggle of loneliness. Yes, our emotions can communicate some positive motivation, like connection or human improvements. However, if we only see the positive in an emotion, we invalidate the difficulties that come with the how and why we feel the emotion. If we only focus on the pain of the emotion, it can be easy to forget that it might be communicating and motivating something important that we need.

In addition, in the field of veterinary medicine, a large part of the day is spent connecting with people you might not feel emotionally connected to. This can create loneliness as well. The people you are working with may feel emotionally connected to you, as you are the person who is saving the animal they are dependent on. However, you may not feel a strong connection to them, as you are focused on the animal and your job. This disconnection can feel confusing to the body and create all kinds of emotions, including loneliness, shame, and disconnection (all of which are often linked together and complicated). The fake connection and sometimes a need to emotionally disconnect to do your job well can create exhaustion toward the connections that we need.

FOOD FOR THOUGHT JOURNALING:

1. Where do you see well-being struggles show up in yourself and around you in the field?

2. How do burnout, compassion fatigue, vicarious trauma, secondary trauma, moral injury, decision-making fatigue, and loneliness show up for you and other colleagues in the field?

3. How can you begin talking about work-related stress in your clinic or setting?

REFERENCES

American Animal Hospital Association (2018). *AAHA's guide to veterinary practice team wellbeing* [White paper]. Available at: https://www.aaha.org/wp-content/uploads/globalassets/04-practice-resources/practice-culture/team_wellbeing_guide.pdf

da Silva, C. R. *et al.* (2023). 'Suicide in veterinary medicine: A literature review', *Veterinary World*, 16(6), pp. 1266–1276. https://doi.org/10.14202/vetworld.2023.1266-1276.

Kulari, G. and Pereira de Castro, M. (2024). 'Depressive symptoms, loneliness and social support in healthcare employees: Does the source of support matter?', *Journal of Public Mental Health*, 23(4), pp. 348–356.

Lecec-Tosevski, D., Vukovic, O. and Stepaniovic, J. (2011). 'Stress and personality', *Psychiatriki*, 22(4), pp. 290–297.

Leris, D. and Byrne, M. K. (2003). 'Vicarious traumatisation: Symptoms and predictors', *Stress and Health*, 19, pp. 129–138. https://doi.org/10.1002/smi.969.

Manning, K. E. *et al.* (2024). 'Merck Animal Health Veterinary Team Study reveals factors associated with wellbeing, burnout, and mental health among nonveterinarian practice team members', *Journal of the American Veterinary Medical Association*, 262(10), pp. 1330–1337. https://doi.org/10.24.0/javma.24.03.0225.

Nashwan, A. J. *et al.* (2024). 'Resilience in solitude: A review of loneliness and its impact on nurses' wellbeing', *Perspectives in Psychiatric Care*, 2024(2024), p. 5225026.

Schaufeli, W. B., De Witte, H., Hakanen, J. J., Kaltiainen, J. and Kok, R. (2023). 'How to assess severe burnout? Cutoff points for the Burnout Assessment Tool (BAT) based on three European samples', *Scandinavian Journal of Work, Environment & Health*, 49(4), pp. 293–302.

Schaufeli, W. B., Desart, S. and De Witte, H. (2020). 'Burnout assessment tool (BAT)—Development, validity, and reliability', *International Journal of Environmental Research and Public Health*, 17(24), 9495.

Stetina, B. U. and Krouzecky, C. (2022). 'Reviewing a decade of change for veterinarians: Past, present and gaps in researching stress, coping and mental health risks', *Animals*, 12(22), 3199. https://doi.org/10.3390/ani12223199.

Strand, E. *et al.* (2017). 'Adverse childhood experiences among veterinary medical students: A multi-site study', *Journal of Veterinary Medical Education*, 44(2), pp. 260–267.

CHAPTER 6

Mental Health in the Veterinary Field

While well-being is a day-to-day struggle for many, mental health goes much deeper than just well-being. Mental health is chronic and more severe. It affects the neurotransmitters in the body and often needs longer, more defined treatment for improvement. While well-being is usually affected by mental health and vice versa, they are separated by these distinctions. Unfortunately, the veterinary field not only struggles with well-being, but there is also a very high rate of mental health struggles in the field. Cases of depression and anxiety are higher among those in the veterinary profession than the rate of others in the general population (da Silva *et al.*, 2023; Smith, Barcelos and Mills, 2023). In fact, in 2023, 1 out of every 11 practitioners with less than 5 years of experience had anxiety and/or depression (da Silva *et al.*, 2023). It is unclear if the high rates of mental health are linked to the well-being related to the field, but it is important to note the prevalence. It can be tempting to say that someone is depressed or anxious or whatever the diagnosis may be. I encourage the language around mental health to change. Saying someone is… can infer that this is who the person is. I prefer to say that someone has symptoms of (whatever diagnosis the person fits the criteria for). While it may feel like it when symptoms are pervasive, you are more than your mental health symptoms.

HOW DO YOU KNOW IF YOU ARE STRUGGLING WITH MENTAL HEALTH?

While work-related stressors like burnout, compassion fatigue, and vicarious trauma can lead to depression, anxiety, and post-traumatic stress disorder (PTSD), and those same mental health symptoms can make one more susceptible to work-related stressors, they can be separated in many ways. Just because someone is sad or burnt out does not mean that they are depressed. Depression, anxiety, and PTSD are all diagnosable in the mental health diagnostic manual (DSM-5) produced by the American Psychiatric Association (2013). The DSM is used by professionals to diagnose, creating a common language for mental health symptoms. However, burnout, compassion fatigue, and vicarious trauma are considered occupational stressors.

There is a growing movement for self-diagnosis, which can be very problematic. There is an influx of people finding a diagnosis on social media. Sometimes this is great and validating and encourages people to get help. The problem becomes when people begin to identify with the diagnosis very strongly. It becomes an identity, and sometimes symptoms occur that were not happening before. While fully self-diagnosing and online researching can be problematic, gathering information and being curious can be very helpful. Knowing that struggles are pervasive, so that one can get the help they need, is necessary for change to happen. If you believe you fit the criteria for a mental health diagnosis, I encourage you to talk with a licensed professional openly so that they can help you decide the appropriate avenue for support and change. Understanding mental health can be important for knowing how to get your own help, and it can also help support others around you.

Just as diagnosing yourself can be a slippery slope, diagnosing others can be equally harmful. Information is not always monitored on the internet, and sometimes blogs, articles, reels, and posts give false information that can lead to inappropriately diagnosing someone in your life. While false diagnoses can be problematic, noticing someone struggling and allowing for support can be validating. Presenting someone with questions can be a great way to discuss struggles you've seen in another person. Saying, "Hey, I know that people can struggle, do you feel like this fits you?" feels much better than saying, "Hey, I think you have...." You can also present this with observation, "I noticed that you are... is everything okay?" This way of communicating with others can open up a conversation that can encourage people to get the help they need.

People mask. They mask to themselves, and they mask to others. Masking refers to the ability to cover up emotions so that a struggle is not seen. Letting people see that things are not going so well can be very vulnerable. People may make a joke about mental health or mention how terrible things are in a passing way, but the reality is that really showing what is going on can be vulnerable and scary. Here is a checklist of things that can be warning signs that you or someone else is not doing well. I developed this list based on personal observation, diagnostic criteria, and well-being assessments. I did not separate diagnosis so that self-diagnosis is not an option. If you mark symptoms and feel ashamed, please know you can't help these symptoms. You may be able to cover them up to an extent, but if you are struggling, they are going to happen whether you like it or not. You are not weak just because you are struggling. There is hope with the appropriate help you need. Keep in mind a person snuggling with a diagnosable mental health disorder will likely mark several of the boxes, not just a few.

- Moving slower

- Decreased interest in activities

- Significant weight loss or weight gain

- Low energy

- Feeling worthless

- Distracting inappropriate guilt every day

- Difficulty thinking and concentrating

- Difficulty in decision-making

- Recurrent thoughts of death or killing yourself

- Difficulty with hygiene

- Restlessness

- Feeling on edge/irritable

- Difficulty falling or staying asleep

- Muscle tension

- Shallow breath

- Wanting to run away

- Excessive worry that is distracting

- Difficulty relaxing
- Feeling a sense of doom
- Excessive worry about your fate or the fate of your loved ones
- Jumpiness
- Hypervigilance
- Wanting to work more
- Wanting to work less
- Dread of most days
- Regular nightmares
- Waking in the middle of the night, thinking about cases
- Feeling disconnected from people around you
- Feeling pessimistic about the future
- Excessive use of substances
- An increase in imposter syndrome (feeling not good enough)
- Difficulty in decision-making
- Feeling disconnected from yourself
- Feeling disconnected from your work
- Feeling grouchy at everything
- Avoiding a specific type of patient
- Feelings are sad most of the time
- Avoiding activities you once enjoyed
- Extreme cynicism
- Avoiding paperwork (if this is not a typical trait)
- Setting healthy routines aside
- Feeling jittery in your body
- Difficulty concentrating
- Feeling grossed out by the positive
- A desire to wallow or sulk
- A feeling of flight from the field
- Impulsiveness

When life becomes more difficult, we may be more vulnerable to mental health conditions. It is as if, as life becomes difficult, your body's default is the mental health diagnoses. Sometimes these symptoms become dormant until life becomes more difficult. Being aware of life stressors that can increase your likelihood of developing mental health symptoms can increase your awareness so that you can get help sooner and stay miserable for less time.

THINGS THAT MAKE YOU MORE VULNERABLE:

- An increase in personal life stressors (shit is hitting the fan)
- A history of trauma
- A history of long-term stress in your environment
- Medical struggles
- Lack of sleep
- Increase in substance use
- It's been a long time since you took an extra day off
- Sedentary lifestyle
- Relationship difficulties
- Change in jobs
- Fatigue
- Cynicism
- Feeling inept
- Lack of positive support
- A Toxic work environment
- Changes in life (a move, new member of the family, etc.)

WHAT SHOULD YOU DO IF YOU BELIEVE YOU MAY HAVE SYMPTOMS OF A MENTAL HEALTH DIAGNOSIS?

If this section is ringing true and you believe that you may fit the criteria for a mental health diagnosis, you must reach out to a mental health professional. This can be a daunting task if you are someone who believes that Mental Health is a weakness. The reality is that mental health comes from an imbalance of neurotransmitters. This can be due to many different factors. Some people are born with a disposition to a mental health concern. Some people have had many things happen in their lives that have created an unsafe body responds in a way that creates an imbalance of neurotransmitters. Some people overuse substances and really do not know how to stop, which can also create this imbalance. It does not exactly matter what created the mental health struggle that you're living with today. What is true is that it can be managed so that you can establish a happy life. I know I can say this a million times, and shame will still exist, but I am going to keep saying it, hoping it will sink in just a little. Therapy, medication, and sometimes alternative treatment such as psychedelic-assisted therapy and Transmagnetic Stimulation can create hope in your life. I know that can be scary, but it can be the difference between living in misery and finding happiness.

When looking for a mental health professional, you must find someone who may be a good fit for you. I encourage you to interview people and see who may connect with you so that you can see hope. Ask questions about their treatment style and make sure it fits your needs. Look at their picture. If you feel like something is off in their picture, you will probably struggle to trust them. We should not judge others by outward appearance, but sometimes we can get a vibe by the way a person looks that can help us find the right fit for therapy. You can find professionals through your insurance, employee assistance programs, directory websites such as Good Therapy or Psychology Today or by asking friends who they are seeing for help. If it feels overwhelming to try to find the perfect fit, pick a random one to start, but if it doesn't work, don't give up, try another one. Mental health is often covered by insurance, which helps with financial concerns. I understand that with a high deductible or a community where few practitioners accept insurance, committing to this kind of help can be a struggle. It is okay to ask for sliding scale practitioners or people who have a scholarship fund so they can help with the finances. There are often ways to receive help, even if it feels like you can't afford it.

Time can also be a barrier. I encourage you to give a limited amount of time to trying therapy if you are overwhelmed by the time. It can feel way too overwhelming to think about setting aside an hour a week for treatment indefinitely. If you give yourself 3 months to set aside an hour a week, this may feel more manageable. Depending on your needs, you may also look into expedited or intensive treatment. Some therapies have been shown to be effective over longer appointment time. You can work through some of your struggles in a full day or a few days, rather than an hour a week. The barrier to this treatment model is that it is rarely covered by insurance.

I wish there were fewer barriers to treatment, but this is the reality of my field. While many clinicians try to be creative to be accessible as possible, I realize there are real barriers to getting therapy for some. In addition to this, we also struggle to prioritize this as a need. We may have the time and money, but we prefer to spend them elsewhere. Therapy can be scary and not always enjoyable. If you are struggling to find a way to make therapy work for you, I encourage you to explore whether your perceived barriers are actually obstacles. If they are, I encourage you to explore the programs available in your community. If they are not actual barriers, please acknowledge that you are using these reasons as excuses more than reasons and set up a plan for making it work, even if it is temporarily uncomfortable. Mental Health symptoms are uncomfortable too, so which one do you choose?

If it feels overwhelming to find mental health support, I encourage you to start at the lowest-hanging fruit for you. If this means calling the Employee Assistance Program with your clinic and saying who do you have available, that is an okay first step. If it means pulling up a directory and emailing the first three you see, that is fine too. Hopefully, that person can point you in the right direction if it is not them. The key here is to know that it is scary and that it is worth it. If nothing else, give it a shot; if it doesn't work, you can always stop.

FOOD FOR THOUGHT JOURNALING:

1. What is scary about addressing my mental health concerns?

2. Where do I see a struggle with well-being and/or mental health show up in my life?

3. What is my plan if I see signs of well-being or mental health struggles in myself?

4. What is my plan if I see signs of well-being or mental health struggles in others?

5. What is scary about addressing concerns with others?

REFERENCES

American Psychiatric Association (2013). *Diagnostic and Statistical Manual of Mental Disorders* (5th ed.). Washington, DC: American Psychiatric Publishing.

da Silva, C. R. *et al.* (2023). 'Suicide in veterinary medicine: a literature review', *Veterinary World*, 16(6), pp. 1266–1276. https://doi.org/10.14202/vetworld. 2023.1266-1276.

Smith, E. T., Barcelos, A. M. and Mills, D. S. (2023). 'Links between pet ownership and exercise on the mental health of veterinary professionals', *Veterinary Record Open*, 10(1), e62. https://doi.org/ 10.1002/vro2.62.

Unhealthy Coping Strategies

CHAPTER 7

ADDICTIVE SUBSTANCES AND BEHAVIORS

While we know that drug and alcohol abuse is higher in stressful environments, and veterinary medicine is a stressful environment, the use of drugs and alcohol is not widely talked about. It is socially acceptable in the field to drink, and there is a great fear of regulatory boards. With the heightened stigma, it becomes a difficult topic (Cormier and Seddon, 2024). If addiction and overuse are spoken of, people may have to stop or reduce their consumption, which is not only hard work but also less fun. I can tell you through discussions with many veterinarians that many veterinarians depend on alcohol to relax their nervous system after a difficult day. Many of those I speak to in the veterinary profession do not consider this a problem, even when drinking in excess is a common practice. Alcohol use is higher among veterinary professionals than in the general population, which makes sense given the higher levels of well-being and mental health concerns (Cormier and Seddon, 2024). High rates of well-being struggles, depression, and suicide are also linked with substance use, making it an important topic to discuss, even though it is difficult (Hernández-Trujillo et al., 2025; Kumar and Saini, 2025; Kieschnick, 2024; Lehnus, Fordyce and McMillan, 2024).

Outside of alcohol, veterinarians also have access to controlled substances that can become addictive. Many veterinary offices have opioids, tranquilizers, and ketamine on hand to be used with animals in need. These are also substances that can be overused by humans. Ensuring controlled substances are properly monitored in a veterinary office is more challenging than one might hope. The fast-paced environment makes safety procedures difficult to abide by. With many veterinary medicines becoming popular street drugs, and the statistics around well-being in the veterinary field being ominous, I can infer that the use of controlled substances is also more prominent than what is discussed. Please keep this in mind when deciding whether it is worth it to maintain safety procedures around controlled substances. Take note when colleagues become more interested in the safety procedures or ask to be alone with the substances. Keep in mind the risks of the drugs in the office.

People use drugs and alcohol to cope because they work in the short term. Dopamine is the neurotransmitter in our brain that is released when we survive as a race. We show spikes of dopamine when we eat, exercise, complete a task, and have sex. However, when we are feeling blue or depressed, our dopamine is depleted. Drugs and alcohol produce a surge of dopamine, which is a fast and effective relief from the difficult. However, when we are not using our drug of choice, we have less dopamine to produce (it was used up in the surge). Our body then communicates a need for the thing that made us feel good, and thus dependency is created (Ma and Zhu, 2014).

Alcohol and drugs are not the only thing that produces this dopamine. Many other non-chemical addictions exist. Some addictions that are common are food, gambling, porn, and the internet. All of these nonchemical addictions produce dopamine in the same way that drugs and alcohol do; however, they are produced due to an action instead of a substance. The internet is the largest growing addiction due to accessibility through cellphones and social media. Just like drugs and alcohol, internet addiction affects performance, sleep, and quality of life. There is a consistent correlation between internet use and high rates of depression and suicide (Hernández-trujillo et al., 2025).

A question I often get is, "When do I know if my use is a problem?" My easy answer is when it negatively impacts your life. The problem here is that it is difficult to self-assess when something that works so well negatively affects your life. The desire to use the substance or perform the behavior exists because it feels good. This makes it difficult to access if it negatively impacts your life. On the surface, it relaxes your nervous system, helps you sleep, and turns off ruminating thoughts. If you look at the surface, no, it does not negatively impact my life; in fact, I should use more because it works so well. The reality is that no amount of skills I teach will work faster and better than substances or addictive behaviors. The problem is what happens below the surface. People tend to isolate when addicted. This isolation fosters bigger feelings of burnout and loneliness. People who once cared for those around them may become more distant due to shame, creating a larger divide in much-needed connections. This isolation can lead to divorce, reduced contact with children, and few, if any, friends. Substances also interfere with the use of lasting coping mechanisms, making the stressors of the day linger in the nervous system. When things linger without being addressed, they accumulate and manifest as irritability, compassion fatigue, burnout, and other struggles. Substances can linger or hangovers can occur, creating a challenge to their effectiveness in your job. Most also create an imbalance of neurotransmitters post-use, increasing symptoms of anxiety and depression.

While substances may seem like they help with sleep, over time, substances such as marijuana and alcohol can reduce the quality of sleep, and it becomes more difficult to sleep without the substance. The sleep is also not quality, leaving someone feeling like they cannot become rested. Most importantly, it is much more likely that you will attempt to take your own life when under the influence of a substance. When under the influence, decision-making is blurred, and people are more likely to be impulsive (Cormier and Seddon, 2024).

So how do you know if your substance use or behavior is out of control when the consequences can be hard to see?

- Are you able to stop use for significant periods of time *comfortably*? (People will often say I give up substances for a month out of the year, I must not be addicted, but if you are gritting your teeth and white-knuckling the whole time, it may still be problematic.)

- Have you tried to reduce or quit without success?

- Do you use substances (perform the behavior) most nights of the week?

- Do you think about and plan using your substance (or acting on the behavior) of choice throughout the day?

- Do you struggle to use your substance (or behavior) of choice in moderation?

- Are you isolating yourself so that you have more time with your substance or behavior?

- Have people around you commented on the use of your substance or behavior?

- Are you irritable when you have not used your substance of choice (or acted on the behavior) in a period of time, or when you are feeling the effects of the substance?

- Can you sleep, socialize, and work as effectiveness as you did before using substances or acting on the behavior?

- Are you hiding the amount of substances you use (or frequency of the behavior) from the people around you?

- As you review these questions, do you notice your brain saying "yes....but"?

- Have you used the substance during the workday to cope or negate withdrawal symptoms?

- Are you extremely uncomfortable with this section of the book, and find yourself justifying your use as you read?

As you review these questions and assess if your substance use is negatively impacting your life, I encourage you to ask family and friends what they think. This can be a very difficult task as it means you are being vulnerable. They might say they believe you have a problem, which would be a huge bummer. They may check in on you and make sure you are doing okay, which would feel uncomfortable. It may also reduce your shame and create a support system. If you think you have a struggle with substance use, please talk to a professional. Quitting on your own is extremely painful. A trained professional can help and make it more realistic and more comfortable (Lehnus, Fordyce and Mcmillan, 2024).

FOOD FOR THOUGHT JOURNAL TOPIC:

1. What is your relationship with substances (coffee, alcohol, marijuana, or controlled substances, internet)? *It may also be helpful to look at other addictions like food, sex, gambling, etc.*

2. What barriers do you have to reducing or quitting substance use? What barriers do you face when discussing it with others?

3. What would you do if you notice increased substance abuse or isolation in others?

4. What emotions come up for you when we discuss substance use and addiction?

OVERWORKING

We feel like we are doing well, we are getting our job done, and working hard. However, working too much can be used as an avoidant strategy and can be problematic over time. Because the nature of the job makes it easy to over-identify with the job, and the struggle with self-compassion and not feeling good enough is common, work can easily become an outlet. It is important to increase your knowledge in the field and grow; however, I often see people spending their night studying the case that did not go well, or gaining more information on something they had to refer out. When this happens too much, it becomes an avoidant strategy that is now an unhealthy coping mechanism. It is less likely for people to express concern for overwork, as it is often expected in the field.

Sometimes, we have to work late to get things done. Sometimes we need to research to gain more information. When it is done frantically and too often, it becomes problematic. Working overtime gives real relief from boredom and isolation. It feels good to get things done and have purpose, but there are real negative side effects to overworking. Exceeding 12 hours of work in a day reduces cognitive performance and efficiency at work, as well as increases cardiovascular risk, high blood pressure, diabetes, and high BMI (Prasad and Thakur, 2019).

For example, early in my career, I received large amounts of training to address my anxiety about being the best therapist I can be. I now receive a large amount of training based on curiosity. It has a different vibe, and I chose my information more carefully. I moved from frantic and avoidant to productive.

Unfortunately, it is common for clinics to take advantage of the passion for the job, the desire to always be better, and the personalities in the field. They praise a desire to work longer hours and dedicate your whole being to your career. Sometimes working less is frowned upon and considered lazy. This perpetuates the positive reinforcement of working as an avoidant strategy.

So what are you avoiding? Many times, people overwork to avoid anxiety. This could be an anxiety that the to-do list is never-ending. It can be anxiety that you do not know enough. Anxiety around making a mistake. There may be messaging about hard work that makes you scared that you will be perceived as lazy. I encourage you to explore the why when you are working long hours several days a week. Is it needed? What would happen if you worked just slightly less? Are you trying to avoid an unavoidable emotion? You work in a fast-paced environment where there is little time to feel and process emotions. This can communicate to your body that working hard is a great way to avoid the sometimes painful process of feeling the emotions in the day.

Sometimes, you are not avoiding work-related emotions; you are avoiding home-related emotions. Home may be lonely and quiet. It may be volatile or have some awkward tension. Maybe it feels more stressful than being at work. It makes sense that you would avoid working too much.

There are times when you need to work late. This may be often. To check if this is destructive, I encourage you to check in and see if you are avoiding something. If you are, please acknowledge that while it may be more comfortable to work right now, avoidance is never permanent, and it is likely whatever you are avoiding will come back bigger and stronger.

If you are working late out of what feels like obligation vs. avoidance, it is important to check in on how it is affecting your life. Are you missing out on other parts of your life? When any part of our identity is overused, we lose sight of other authentic parts of ourselves. This leads to value deficits, burnout, and other work-related stress responses. No matter what your reason for overworking is, the side effects are the same: increased risk for mental health concerns and physical health concerns (Prasad and Thakur, 2019).

There is always work that can be done. The to-do list will never be accomplished. You will never have all the knowledge possible. It is okay to establish some limits with yourself about when to be uncomfortable, even when there is still work to be done. You have to decide what a reasonable limit is. It is different in all situations.

FOOD FOR THOUGHT JOURNAL TOPIC:

1. When I work after hours, am I avoiding anything?

2. Does the amount that I work get in the way of other parts of my life?

3. What is my plan moving forward? Is this realistic? What can I do to make it realistic?

ISOLATION

I often meet veterinarians who leave work and go home to their pet and a desire not to talk to anyone. This makes sense to me, after talking to wonderful and less-than-wonderful humans all day, especially if you tend to be an introvert. This in itself is a healthy, effective coping mechanism. What is not a healthy mechanism is when this becomes exaggerated, and there are no people outside of your clinic whom you talk to. It perpetuates a feeling that people do not understand you and that your job (which has moments of yuck) is all that you are. It can feel like no one outside of veterinarians themselves understands veterinarians. I encourage you to challenge yourself to connect with humans several times a week. If they are other veterinarians because this is more comfortable, that is fine. I encourage you to make a rule that you are not allowed to talk about work. You will probably talk about work some, but the rule can allow for more topics as well. The connections I am encouraging do not have to be a deep connection. If it is difficult to connect through deep conversation, you can connect by getting your groceries in person so that you have to smile at the cashier, try a hobby that has a group aspect to it, go for a walk in a busy park, and say hi to a person you walk by. This small amount of human interaction can create a level of connectedness outside of the veterinary office that can remind you that there is more to the world than what you see within the clinic.

FOOD FOR THOUGHT JOURNALING:

1. Check in with yourself. Do you find yourself isolation to avoid? Is it effective in the long run?

2. Notice any desire to avoid connection. What is isolation protecting from? What is your fear?

REFERENCES

American Psychiatric Association (2013). *Diagnostic and Statistical Manual of Mental Disorders* (5th ed.). Washington, DC: American Psychiatric Publishing.

Cormier, O. and Seddon, J. (2024). 'Alcohol-related stigma within the UK veterinary profession', *Veterinary Record*, 195(9), e4532.

Hernández-Trujillo, I. *et al.* (2025). 'Psychological well-being, substance use, and internet consumption among students and teaching staff of the Faculty of Veterinary Medicine: Risk and protective factors associated with well-being and dissatisfaction', *Healthcare (Basel)*, 13(8), p. 918. MDPI.

Kieschnick, D. (2024). 'Veterinary Medicine and Substance Use.' *dvm360*, 55(5), p. 48.

Kumar, K. and Saini, S. S. (2025). 'The lethal mix: Substance abuse and suicidal behaviour', in Kumar, U. (ed.) *Handbook of Suicide Prevention: Insights, Strategies and Approaches.* Singapore: Springer Nature Singapore, pp. 329–352.

Lehnus, K. S., Fordyce, P. S. and McMillan, M. W. (2024). 'Electronic survey investigating UK veterinarians' perceptions of the potential for veterinary prescription medication misuse or abuse', *Veterinary Anaesthesia and Analgesia*, 51(1), pp. 16–25.

Ma, H. and Zhu, G. (2014). 'The dopamine system and alcohol dependence', *Shanghai Archives of Psychiatry*, 26(2), pp. 61–68. https://doi.org/10.3969/j.issn.1002.0829.2014.02.002.

Prasad, B. and Thakur, C. (2019). 'Chronic overworking: Cause extremely negative impact on health and quality of life', *International Journal of Advanced Microbiology and Health Research*, 3(1), pp. 11–15.

CHAPTER 8

Suicide

It is with a heavy heart that I acknowledge that we cannot talk about mental health in the veterinary field without talking about suicide. It is likely that you know someone or know someone who knows someone in the field who has successfully taken their own life. Suicide professionals often say high rates of suicide among specific populations are due to a means. This holds true in the veterinary profession, with the most common way that people kill themselves being poisoning, followed by firearms (da Silva *et al.*, 2023). Those in the veterinarian profession are four times more likely to kill themselves than the general population and twice as likely as those in other healthcare professions (Smith, Barcelos and Mills, 2023; Smits *et al.*, 2023). Since 1999, statistics of suicide being higher than the general population have been shown in the veterinary field and have continued to increase every 5 years (Tomasi *et al.*, 2019). This leads me to wonder, why are suicide rates so high, and why are they increasing? The continued increase suggests that the stigma surrounding this ongoing struggle has plagued this profession for many years (Ho *et al.*, 2023). While this is a heavy, scary topic, it is essential to discuss.

PREVENTION

The first step in suicide prevention is to develop a plan. With suicide statistics being so heartbreaking in the field, you will likely encounter some type of suicide crisis in your career. Developing a plan before it happens can ensure you respond effectively and with less frantic, anxious energy. It is important to take all talk about suicide seriously, even if it is said in passing or as a joke. Contrary to popular belief, it is uncommon for people to threaten to kill themselves for attention. Please listen when people talk about killing themselves. One person caring can make a difference.

People tend to use what is most available to them to kill themselves, and even if the plan is carefully thought out, the actual act is often done impulsively. This means that the best way to help people stop killing themselves is to make the means less easy to access. While many laws protect restricted medications, someone always holds the key to the medication closet. If there is a practice rule that no one is allowed in the medication closet without a companion, it is easy to let this slide when people get busy (da Silvia et al., 2023). I encourage you to follow the Drug Enforcement Administration guidelines to the best of your ability, limiting access to drugs that someone could use in suicide. You may also increase safety with additional lock boxes and time-lapsed locks, increasing the time it takes to access lethal means. I know that this is inconvenient, but if we want to save some lives, we need to acknowledge that this is a problem within the field and take it very seriously, even when it is far from convenient. There's a common misconception that many of the reasons that suicide is so high in veterinary medicine is because of the option for euthanasia and pets. The research shows that euthanasia often creates relief when a pet is suffering, and there is no correlation between euthanasia and suicidality. However, with euthanasia medication often on-site at a veterinary office, there is a link between access to a very lethal means and success in suicide (Cooney and Kipperman, 2023; Smits, 2022).

We must break the stigma of talking about suicide. Just because you avoid talking about something does not make the problem go away. Talking about suicide and suicide prevention openly creates more space for people to talk about their struggles. People are more likely to connect with someone open about a topic because that person is more likely to be better at listening to the topic (da Silvia et al., 2023). Yes, it is uncomfortable, but it is essential to ask people who seem to be having a difficult time if they want to kill themselves.

What we know about suicide is that it is contagious. Knowing someone who has killed themselves makes it much more likely that you will follow through as well (Smits, 2022). When assessing someone for risk for suicide, knowing someone who has attempted or successfully killed themselves is a significant risk factor. It is unknown why exactly suicide holds this power, but it can give someone who has been thinking about it the courage to follow through, or it may even give someone an idea who is feeling stuck in their current struggle. Whatever the reason for the contagion, it does communicate that if we can reduce suicide in the field even a little, we must talk about it and address it in teams when it happens. It also communicates that we need to check on people who have someone close to them who has taken their life. Let these people know they are important.

When we identify and support people who are at risk of suicide, the harm is reduced (Tomasi *et al.*, 2019). The Center for Discease Control reports (2022) seven strategies for managing suicide. Among these strategies, supporting access to suicidal care is one. This can be done by ensuring Employment Assisted Programs (EAP) and access to therapy are available to all employees of veterinary clinics. It is also encouraged to promote connection and teach coping strategies. This can be done during schooling or within clinics. When people are struggling, it can be helpful to have information about coping strategies available. This could be pamphlets created by a local clinic or posters with quick coping mechanisms around the clinic. Lastly, promoting connection is essential for suicide prevention. Creating space and encouraging connection are essential in this process (Tomasi *et al.*, 2019). In order to take the steps toward preventing suicide, we need to address the problem more than mentioning it in passing. Veterinarians need to know how to assess for risk factors, support those around them, and limit means. I want to be clear, you are not the only one responsible for the lives of everyone around you. It is simply important to be comfortable with conversations and know basic risk factors so that you can refer people to services when it is necessary. While more support is given and more nonprofits are forming to address this concern, there is still a large part of the field that is turning a blind eye to suicide risks in the field.

HOW DO YOU TALK TO PEOPLE ABOUT SUICIDE?

I have listed all the reasons we need to begin openly and honestly talking about suicide within the profession of veterinary medicine, but the biggest question is how. It can be terrifying to talk to people about killing themselves, and there is a common misconception that if you talk about it, you will give people the idea to follow through. It can also be uncomfortable if you are worried about making the person uncomfortable. The reality is that openly talking about suicide reduces the risk and increases the likelihood that someone will get the help they need to stay alive (Stoewen, 2015). The worst-case scenario is that the person has no intention of killing themselves, and now they know that you care enough about them to want them to be alive. It is essential to ask people directly if you are concerned. Asking indirect questions like, "Are you okay?" or "Do you need anything?" is much less effective than directly asking, "I see you are struggling. Do you want to kill yourself?" If the answer is no, then great. Maybe the person will feel seen for their struggle and get the help they need in whatever way they feel comfortable. If the answer is yes, you can support the person and get them the help they need.

Asking about suicide also shows that people care about the person, reducing loneliness, and a belief that people will be better off if they are dead.

It is very important to take all suicide talk seriously. Research shows that people who attempt suicide are very likely to have mentioned their desire to others, even if in a sarcastic, seemingly harmless way (Stowen, 2015). You may be thinking, "Gosh, it is a lot of work to call out every person who has mentioned wanting to kill themselves on a bad day." Taking all talk seriously can reduce this type of banter and create a more serious perspective on suicide. Without taking suicide seriously, we cannot address the very real problem, and we cannot save lives.

If you know someone who has attempted suicide and stayed alive, it is important to take this attempt seriously. A person who has attempted suicide is more likely to try again without the appropriate support. It is important not to respond with, "Aren't you glad you stayed alive?" Because this may not be true for that person. You can rephrase this: "I am glad you are alive; how can I support you moving forward." Unfortunately, suicide attempts are often seen as a cry for help when they need serious support and professional assistance.

If you are scared of conversations about death, please practice having these difficult conversations with a colleague. This can help you be more confident when the skill is needed.

RISK FACTORS IN SUICIDE

Many risk factors contribute to an increased thought of killing oneself. Knowing these risk factors can give you the knowledge to support someone in need. While depression is often a symptom someone may experience before suicide, a sudden improvement is also an indicator of suicide risk. The person may have been so debilitated by depression that they did not have the energy to take the action to kill themselves, and when they improve slightly, they have the energy to follow through. The person may also have an improved mood because they have decided to follow through and feel hope in their current situation when death is an option. This does not mean that everyone happy is at risk of suicide. The risk falls when someone is very depressed and suddenly is not depressed and has large amounts of energy.

Recklessness and drinking are also indicators that someone is at risk for suicide. Even if death by suicide is planned out, the actual act is often impulsive and inhibited by substances.

Many times, people expect someone to write a letter or withdraw when they are planning suicide. This is true sometimes; however, it is more likely that the person will begin calling and visiting people they love. They begin to say goodbye without actually saying the words. They crave comfort for their loved one's future grief.

A person planning to kill themselves will often begin to give away possessions so that they know that someone will take care of their things. Maybe they start finalizing their will, paying into or canceling life insurance, or discussing how their animal will be cared for if they are not present. The person may also become more interested in the medication cabinet. They may begin discussing safety procedures in a curious detail, ask where the keys are kept, or request permission to enter without a colleague (Tomasi et al., 2019). The person may acquire a gun or some other deadly means to prepare for their suicide.

If you notice any of these risk factors, please speak with the person compassionately and directly about your concerns immediately. Have suicide prevention resources available and practice the conversations ahead of time. If you miss the risk factors, or someone kills themselves despite your efforts to intervene, it can create grief, shame, and self-blame. Please know that you did what you could to save their life. Unfortunately, not everyone can be saved. While it is important to have the skills and abilities to talk about and prevent death by suicide, it is not your responsibility to save every life.

COMMUNICATION WITH STAFF ABOUT SUICIDE

When someone associated with your clinic kills themselves, it is important to be mindful of the language you use. For many years, we discussed taking one's life as committing suicide. This is now considered a harmful phrase as it infers they did something wrong (similar to committing a crime). It also implies that they were obligated to kill themselves. Verbiage like "killed themselves," "took their own life," or "took too many drugs" is a more appropriate way to communicate this difficult topic.

We need to understand that many people do not want to actually die; they are simply in so much pain that they do not see another way to find happiness. Suicide is the ultimate avoidance. Establishing hope for others is essential when discussing suicide. If someone in your clinic dies by suicide, it is imperative to begin being mindful of the other staff's reactions. If they present with more warning signs, it is important to address them immediately, breaking the cycle of death as soon as possible.

It can be helpful to ask local crisis counselors and people trained in emergency response to help with your clinic's conversation and grief. People trained in this conversation can be found through Human Resource organizations, community mental health centers, or local mental health agencies.

Openly acknowledging the risk factors for suicide within your clinic is very important. This can reduce the stigma of talking about this very real topic and increase the likelihood that people will get support as needed. When we speak openly about the issue, we have more people available for support when needed. While this can be intimidating, I strongly encourage the conversation. It does not have to take much time. It can be discussed periodically during staff meetings or during the hiring process. Building a culture around support is essential in saving lives.

WHAT DO I DO IF SOMEONE SAYS THEY WANT TO KILL THEMSELVES?

You are not a mental health professional or expected to be a professional in this situation. You will need to assist the person struggling by contacting someone who can address their needs directly. In the United States, you can call or text 988 to receive assistance for yourself or someone else in crisis. If they are willing, you may drive the person to an emergency room where a professional can assess them. You may also call suicide prevention resources in your area. Having these resources researched and ready to present as needed can be very helpful.

It can feel like a person in a mental health crisis is just one more thing in your busy workday. It can feel annoying and cumbersome. That is okay. Please allow for the time with this person, even if you are annoyed. It is important that you not leave a person who is actively suicidal alone until sufficient support has been given. Call a colleague in to assist if you need to leave to make a call or get resources. You may need to discuss a safety plan with the struggling individual. This would look like having a loved one or trusted friend pick them up from work and be with them. Discuss with them who the safest person in their life may be, so as not to infringe on privacy more than is needed.

It is essential in these situations that suicide and mental health crises not be used in a pejorative way. This person is struggling for a reason, and it is crucial to give them space to suffer and gain the support they need without repercussions from their place of work.

WHAT IF I WANT TO KILL MYSELF?

Please reach out for support. This can be by calling or texting 988, contacting a mental health professional in your area, or telling a trusted friend or mentor. You do not have to suffer with these thoughts alone. If you are concerned about being hospitalized or perceived differently, it is essential to be upfront and honest about this so that the person can explain the steps clearly. If you know the means you would like to use to kill yourself, please ensure that these means are difficult to access. Letting people know you cannot be left alone with medication, asking others to care for a firearm, having someone else temporarily distribute your drugs, or distancing yourself from other lethal means is essential in giving yourself space to receive the help you need. If nothing else, I ask that you try some resources with a shot to see if they may work to alleviate your pain. Without trying to see if they will work, it is impossible to know if they work.

FOOD FOR THOUGHT JOURNAL TOPIC:

1. What feels intimidating about discussing suicide? How can I work through this and address it anyway?

2. What would I do if I learned that a colleague wants to kill themselves?

3. What would be the most challenging part of this plan for me?

4. What would get in the way of me carrying out this plan?

REFERENCES

Centers for Disease Control and Prevention (2022). *Suicide Prevention Resource for Action: A Compilation of the Best Available Evidence*. Atlanta, GA: National Center for Injury Prevention and Control.

Cooney, K. and Kipperman, B. (2023). 'Ethical and practical considerations associated with companion animal euthanasia', *Animals*, 13(3), 430. https://doi.org/10.3390/ani13030430.

da Silva, C. R. *et al.* (2023). 'Suicide in veterinary medicine: A literature review', *Veterinary World*, 16(6), pp. 1266–1276. https://doi.org/10.14202/vetworld.2023.1266-1276.

Ho, N. T., Santoro, F., Palacios Jimenez, C. and Pelligand, L. (2023). 'Cross-sectional survey of sleep, fatigue and mental health in veterinary anaesthesia personnel', *Veterinary Anaesthesia and Analgesia*, 50(4), pp. 315–324. https://doi.org/10.1016/j.vaa.2023.03.003.

Smith, E. T., Barcelos, A. M. and Mills, D. S. (2023). 'Links between pet ownership and exercise on the mental health of veterinary professionals', *Veterinary Record Open*, 10(1), e62. https://doi.org/10.1002/vro2.62.

Smits, F., Houdmont, J., Hill, B. and Pickles, K. (2023). 'Mental wellbeing and psychosocial working conditions of autistic veterinary surgeons in the UK', *Veterinary Record*, 193(8), e3311 https://doi.org/10.1002/vetr.3311.

Smits, F. (2022). *Autistic veterinary surgeons in the United Kingdom: Workplace stressors and mental wellbeing* [Master of Research Thesis, University of Nottingham]. Available at: http://eprints.nottingham.ac.uk/78517/1/14324658_Femke%20Smits_MRES%20thesis%20corrections.pdf

Stoewen, D. L. (2015). 'Suicide in veterinary medicine: let's talk about it.' *The Canadian Veterinary Journal*. 56(1), pp. 89–92. PMID: 25565722; PMCID: PMC4266064.

Tomasi, S. E., Fechter-Leggett, E. D., Edwards, N. T., Reddish, A. D. and Nett, R. J. (2019). 'Suicide among veterinarians in the United States from 1979 through 2015', *Journal of the American Veterinary Medical Association*, 254(1), pp. 104–112. https://doi.org/10.2460/javma.254.1.104.

Barriers to Treatment

CHAPTER 9

ADDRESSING BARRIERS

There are barriers to treating mental well-being and mental health. Without addressing the barriers to care, it is easy to continue feeling stuck and hopeless in the process.

People often attempt to solve a problem without awareness of the whole picture. When we are in distress, we often focus solely on the distressing aspects of the event. This is a protective mechanism in our system. If we do not focus on the aspect of our environment that is causing us pain, we may miss a way to stay safe. This makes logical sense, but it often is more complicated than this. Focusing on the negative leaves us feeling like we are pushing up against a brick wall that will never move. Through awareness, we can see things more effectively and ultimately make moves toward genuine change. This does not mean you look at only the positive. This toxic positivity is also a barrier. The whole picture, both good and bad, is essential to make changes.

Money is a significant barrier to receiving the treatment that is needed for well-being. Access to therapy, well-being discussions, and coaching can be extremely expensive (Dickson, 2023). I recommend looking into a therapist on your insurance or employee assistance program network if it is available. If this is still outside of your financial reach, it may be more beneficial to look into sliding-scale assistance in your community. Sliding scale refers to programs that will assess income and charge based on what people can afford. You may also ask a local therapist if they offer scholarships, as this is available in some communities. If none of these are available to you, I recommend diving deep into whatever self-help speaks to you. There are many podcasts, books, and free CE events that speak to your needs. Following your own path is extremely challenging at times because accountability and outside insights are not as available. It may be beneficial to join with a few trusted peers to review insights and learning to address this accountability. While the most effective way to address concerns is with a licensed mental health professional, I encourage you to start in whatever way is accessible to you.

Time is another significant barrier to addressing well-being needs. This is ironic because time is often the reason for struggles with well-being. It's enough to make your head spin. I recommend having a scheduled time where you can address the needs of your well-being. Sometimes this means going to therapy, journaling, or reading this book. I know all too well that this is easier said than done. When I have to decide whether to relax in bed or do my self-exploration work, relaxing in bed is more likely to win. Sometimes work, kids, and life just get busy, and this is the first thing that drops. It is important to acknowledge when you do let these things drop and redevelop a routine. The busy parts of life will be difficult to manage if you are not addressing your well-being and mental health. As hard as it is, changes need to be a priority. It will be worth it. If you aren't quite sure if you believe me, try to prioritize it for 2–3 weeks.

It is also important to be realistic. If you prefer in-person mental health treatment, but including drive time adds too much time and makes it that much harder to go, you may have to create some flexibility and look into a therapist who offers video platforms. If one hour a week is overwhelming to you, ask your therapist if they would be willing to see you less often. Intensive or expedited therapy may also be an option for those struggling with making time for therapy. This is a model of therapy where people are seen in chunks of time (a day or several days in a row) to work through large amounts of material at once. If all of this feels too overwhelming, think about creating 10 minutes a day to start working on your well-being as a more realistic model. If you are not following through with your plan, it is likely too big, and I encourage you to scale it back. This creates steps that can lead to the ultimate goal.

In a world of easy access to information, there is often too much information, which can become overwhelming. When people first begin to explore well-being and mental health, they sometimes dive in deep to the information. They listen to all the podcasts, read all the books, and surround themselves with wellness. This is great, I do not want to discourage it even a little. However, I also notice that sometimes people use gaining information as a distraction technique for actually working on the stuff. A sports coach of mine used to say, "You can overdose (OD) on Vitamin C." The saying refers to the idea that you can overdo a good thing and it can become destructive. It is so easy to gain information about well-being and mental health; it can be like drinking water from a fire hose. There is so much information out there, all of it coming from separate viewpoints and directions. Some will fit your needs and some will not. I encourage you to try stuff out as if you are throwing darts at a dart board (in an unskilled way), curious what will stick. If it doesn't work, try something else. Be cautious of gaining too much information. Self-help can become a form of avoidance. Some of the information given can have a "rara," feel-good vibe to it, which can allow people to feel good in the short term. I encourage you to explore information with a desire to add one thing to your life that you learn. Practice adding that thing to your life for a week or two before adding more information to the mix.

Unrealistic expectations are also a barrier to change. If you do not follow through, be curious about how realistic the goal is. Either make your goal smaller or change it up in a way that you will follow through. Be realistic with your goal. If the one thing you take away is that you need to spend hours a day meditating, and you have never even tried it, it may not be very realistic.

Motivation is also a barrier to creating space for your well-being. Depression comes with lack of motivation, burnout comes with lack of motivation, and exhaustion comes with lack of motivation. When we are suffering, our neurotransmitters become out of balance. It is the body's way of communicating that we are not getting what we need. It simply becomes an imbalance in the confusion and layers of our thoughts, beliefs, and actions that have been shaped by the life we have lived up until this point. Maybe you really want to do the things to make you feel better, but it feels like climbing Mount Everest. The struggle is REAL. I highly recommend starting small. If you are not achieving your goal, make it smaller until that becomes doable, and move to the next one. Find the small space where you can do something, whether you want to or not. This creates some space for more things to happen. Challenging yourself, no matter how small that challenge may be, creates different neurotransmitters, which over time can create an increase in motivation. Making change possible.

Think about a ladder reaching to the top of a building. If the ladder has no rungs, you probably won't go very far. The more rungs you have, the less you will have to struggle to climb the ladder, and the more likely you are to get to the top. The top of the ladder is where you would like to be. Some people call this the goal or the intention. The steps in the ladder are the steps you need to take. As you can see in Figure 9.1, if they are too far apart, you may become stuck and unable to move. Creating more rungs may feel like a step back, but it is actually creating more rungs to make it more likely that you will get to the top.

I often notice people's Belief system around what it means to ask for help and who asks for help as a barrier to treatment. It is easy to think that going to therapy means that you are broken. I have also heard people say, "My problems are not big enough for therapy" or something along those lines. Another statement I often hear is "What will I have to talk about?" It is important to address expectations for receiving therapy. Each therapeutic style is slightly different, and it is essential to find a therapeutic style that resonates with you and your specific needs. Therapy can be helpful for any level of struggle that you are unable to resolve on your own or don't want to

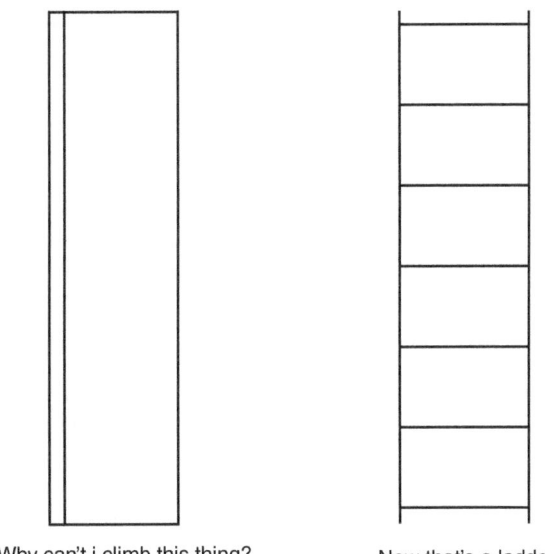

Why can't i climb this thing?   Now that's a ladder

FIGURE 9.1 Two ladders. One with rungs and one without rungs. This depicts the need to make small steps toward change.

resolve on your own. It can help you through more challenging times and miserable times. Sometimes, only a few sessions are needed to ensure you can live the life you need; sometimes, many sessions are required to work through the necessary changes. I encourage you to try out three to six sessions to see what it may be like. Allow the therapist to decide if this is "big enough" for therapy. The answer is likely yes, because therapy can help in a variety of different ways. In addition, you are not broken. There is not a human on this planet who has not gone through a period of their life that is difficult. Our body responds to stress with safety responses. It is doing what it is supposed to do; it is just doing it a little too well. You do not have to figure it out on your own, nor will you be able to, because you are the one living it (Andrade *et al.*, 2014; Ebert *et al.*, 2019).

The largest barrier to treatment is the ongoing stigma of mental health. Because it is taboo to talk about struggles with each other, people often feel like they are the only one struggling. It can feel weak to make the effort to make changes in your life. With simple psychoeducation about mental health, well-being, and avenues to change, people make more changes to improve their well-being (Gannon *et al.*, 2024). It can be tempting to believe that talking about a problem can perpetuate the problem, but the more we talk about the struggles in the field, the more validating it can feel to people in the field. They are likely to feel less alone. If people discuss ways in which they have created positive changes in their lives, people are more likely to make the changes needed to improve their well-being.

FOOD FOR THOUGHT JOURNAL TOPIC:

1. What are my personal barriers that get in the way of my well-being?

2. What steps do I need to take to work past my barriers so that I can live the best life I can live?

3. What is my plan for when I get stuck in my goals? How do I recognize when I'm stuck, and how do I create space to adjust the steps toward my goal?

4. What are my beliefs about well-being (not just what you say out loud, but what you truly believe in your core self)? How might my beliefs contribute to or hinder my journey toward positive well-being?

REFERENCES

Andrade, L. H. *et al.* (2014). 'Barriers to mental health treatment: Results from the WHO World Mental Health surveys', *Psychological Medicine*, 44(6), pp. 1303–1317.

Dickson, B. (2023) *Ethical dilemmas and moral distress in companion animal veterinary medicine: Mental health implications.*/https://scholars.wlu.ca/cgi/viewcontent.cgi?article=3771&context=etd

Ebert, D. D. *et al.* (2019). 'Barriers of mental health treatment utilization among first-year college students: First cross-national results from the WHO World Mental Health International College Student Initiative', *International Journal of Methods in Psychiatric Research*, 28(2), e1782.

Gannon, K. R. *et al.* (2024). 'Exploration of mental health stigma in veterinary teams in the United States before and after evidence-based psychoeducation for burden transfer', *Veterinary Record Open*, 11(2), e84.

Nervous System

It can be very easy to ignore the reactions that our nervous system has throughout the day. We get caught up in the stressors of the day and only notice that our body system is reacting when it is reacting in a major way, like with a panic attack or extreme distress. Our body is actually reacting to situations throughout the day with the intention of finding safety. Just like a seed is constantly trying to find light to grow, our body is always trying to find safety to thrive. Many times we develop natural coping strategies that help us get through difficult situations. Unfortunately, sometimes after these coping mechanisms word our system gets excited and starts overusing them. This is when we have symptoms that are difficult to manage. For instance, maybe your family of origin had several children. You often were ignored due to the need to care for everyone else. However, when you yelled about something everyone saw and heard you. This was very helpful in the moment. As an adult you continue to yell when you feel like you are not seen or heard. It is no longer helpful and causes problems in your relationships. Without knowing this came from something that worked in the past it is hard to create change. When we start to understand our nervous system responses and notice how our own personal system responds we often have the space to thrive and grow in a different way. This section of the book with review how your nervous system works. It will also tie the nervous system to work place stressors. We will then review how to address nervous system responses in order to find safety in the body and reduce the symptoms that make work difficult.

CHAPTER 10

Your Nervous System

WHY THE BRAIN?

Our brains are hardwired for safety. However, it is still very primitive, dating back to the time of saber-tooth tigers. Some days I call it lazy, other days, efficient. In fact, it is so efficient that it is always looking for an easy solution, which may or may not exist. Our brain utilizes patterns that we needed in the past and re-purposes them for what we need today. For instance, the brain figured out a way to find our way back to food sources and our babies, utilizing the firing of specific neurons to anticipate what to expect in day-to-day life. Our body knows how to come back to the things we need to survive as a human race (O'connor, 2022). We may not be able to get to the grocery store without a navigation system, but we do know how to keep things as predictable as possible. Whether you look at trauma studies, grief studies, or people exploring the best way to learn and teach, they all say the same thing: our neural networks are all linked to our primitive and basic instinct to survive. So how the heck does that relate to the day-to-day life of a veterinarian? Everything. You have a lot of expectations going into the career. Heck, there is expectation in every day of our lives. When these expectations are based on curiosity, connection, or maybe some other driver that brought you into the field, that is the neurotransmitter firing. When this expectation is not met, and handlers, animals, and even the system respond differently than your expectation, different neurotransmitters fire, or sometimes none at all. Your thoughts start to expect the worst, become pessimistic, and feel unsafe.

You do not have control over any of this. It is below the level of consciousness. We try really hard to make shifts in our lives by pile-driving through these reactions and telling them to stop. We get mad at ourselves and feel guilty when the reactions keep happening, even though we know it is not the best way. This is because the neuropathways are instinctual, not thought-related. They developed through a series of patterns that have helped us survive as a human race. Our primary drive is to survive above all else. Our brain is going to respond based on this desire to survive more than it will to any of our thoughts. Our neuronetwork, which responds to safety in the world, defines our predator as specific thoughts, emotions, and perceptions. It believes these things will kill us, even though our thoughts know it will not actually kill us.

This is what we are going to dive into in this section of the book. You will learn what is happening in day-to-day life that makes things difficult, how your neurotransmitters respond to these day-to-day interactions, and how to manage them in a way that you can build a safe neuropathway. Easy right? Your nervous system is a driving force in how you manage situations as they present themselves. Because these responses are on the outside of the line of consciousness, they are difficult to address without understanding why we respond the way we do from a deeper level. As you gain a deeper understanding of your reactions, you learn how to work with your system from this perspective, and you gain resilience by working with your nervous system instead of fighting with it. As you become more aware of your own nervous system responses, you may also be able to recognize other people's nervous system responses as well. This can allow more space for empathy, connection, and effective communication with those around you.

POLYVAGAL THEORY

The polyvagal theory has gained popularity, and I would be remiss not to give an overview of the theory in this section. Developed by Stephen Porges in 1994, the basic concept of the theory is that our vagus nerve has three sections. Some people refer to these as our three brains. A quick reminder of the human nervous system helps us understand the concepts of the polyvagal system. Your vagus nerve starts in the cervical area of your spine (around your neck) and runs through your body to your stomach and out to your limbs. Its job is to respond to danger efficiently. This nerve is part of the autonomic nervous system and is how we react spontaneously. The autonomic nervous system is controlled by the amygdala in the brain, a small section located near the start of the vagus nerve. The amygdala cannot function at full capacity when the frontal cortex is at full capacity, and vice versa. This is because the autonomic nervous system is quicker, and when in danger, our body wants the fastest response. The more the amygdala fires, the less the frontal cortex is working. If a bear is eating food out of your refrigerator while you are sitting in the living room, and someone asks you what $2+2$ is, you will probably use some expletives to let them know that math is not important right now and we need to stay safe. The vagus is not just in the autonomic nervous system; it also has ties to the sympathetic nervous system. The sympathetic nervous system is located in the middle of the spinal column and prepares us for action. It is a part of our nervous system that produces adrenaline to protect us from danger. The vagus nerve has two directions in which it can go. Up, which would be into our faces, throat, and ears, this part supports feelings of safety and social connection. The other part moves down and responds to cues of extreme danger. The polyvagal theory hypothesizes that the vagus nerve splits into three separate sections. The three sections of the vagus nerve response are the dorsal vagal, ventral vagal, and the sympathetic nervous system. The dorsal vagal system is the freeze response in simple terms. Simply put, the sympathetic nervous system is the fight or flight, and the ventral vagal system is the connection and safety. The dorsal vagal nerve can be found from below the diaphragm to the bottom of the digestive system, the sympathetic nervous system can be found from the bottom of the diaphragm to the top of the esophagus, and the ventral nervous system can be found in the face.

According to the polyvagal theory, the three sections are based on evolutionary adaptations. The dorsal vagal would be the oldest of the systems coming from our reptilian ancestors. These animals are more likely to freeze when threatened by a predator. The sympathetic would be the next to develop. Our ancestors learned that fighting or running from predators is sometimes more protective than freezing. Lastly, the ventral nervous system was designed with a perceived safety that may not have been available to our early ancestors as they tried to survive. It may also contribute to a pack animal mentality where we connect, respect, and protect each other in our herd.

According to Stephen Porges and his followers, by recognizing our responses and utilizing the three brains or sections of our nervous system and their reactions, we can treat these reactions and find safety. When we define our system in the dorsal, sympathetic, and ventral vagal systems, we can move out of fear responses more easily and start to find safety. For instance, Porges suggests that when we are in a shutdown or freeze response of the dorsal, we may create small movements that can transition us into the sympathetic nervous system. In the sympathetic nervous system, we may generate more intention in our movement, allowing our body to enter the safe and connected ventral vagal system. According to this theory, the heart rate is a significant indicator of which section of the system you are in. A slowed heart rate would indicate a dorsal vagal response, an increased heart rate would indicate a sympathetic response, and a neutral and even heart rate would indicate a ventral vagal.

Porges uses the word "neuroseption" to describe a person's ability to assess for danger without conscious thought. Some refer to this as the "gut feeling." It relates to our ability to take in information from our organs and the environment around us to assess safety. We do not always know that our body is assessing for danger; it is often a subconscious act. Neuroception is not only an assessment of ourselves and our environment; it also refers to the body's ability to access cues in the body language of those around us. It can misalign with our conscious thought when our brain tells us we are safe, but our body reacts with one of the safety responses.

Porges explains the three sections of the vagus nerve as if they were a ladder. One cannot skip rungs and go from a dorsal state to a ventral state of safety. Instead, one must go through all parts of the nervous system to find safety. If one is in a dorsal vagal state, they must pass through the sympathetic nervous system to find safety in the ventral vagal system. I see this often when working with a depressed person. They feel shut down or stuck, and as we work through safety within this system, they become very anxious or want to end the session early. When we work through this section, the person can feel more comfortable and safe. This also happens when someone is very anxious and jittery. The body becomes tired of being in this state and cannot find the safety to move into the ventral vagus nerve, so it gives up and moves to the dorsal vagus nerve (Porges, 2022, 2023) (Figure 10.1).

Here is an example of how the polyvagal system is seen in day-to-day life:

You wake up, notice your alarm did not go off, and you are late. You immediately jump into the sympathetic nervous system, frantically getting ready and rushing out the door to work. You need this frantic state to hustle enough to get out the door on time. There is a safety response here, as you need a job to have financial safety. You remain in the sympathetic nervous system as you rush to work. Someone cuts you off in traffic, and you become outraged as you are already in this response. When you get to work, your boss says "you are late again. Next time, I will have to write you up". This makes you angry, too, but your body struggles to find safety in the sympathetic nervous system, so it moves down to the dorsal vagal system. You feel mopey, move a little slower, and just want to go home and hide. You feel stuck in your life and your job. You may have thoughts of

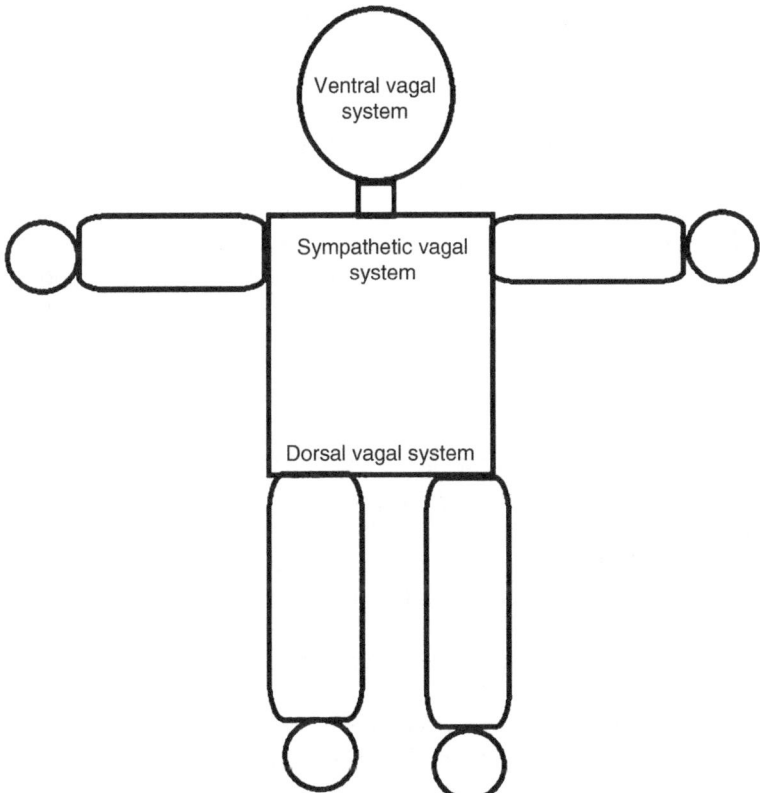

FIGURE 10.1 Showing where each of the sections of the polyvagal system can be seen in the body.

giving up. Your friend comes up to you and says, "What's up with you today." You start complaining about your morning, the bad drivers, and your boss. You get angry and frantic again as you talk about it. It starts to complete itself as you speak with your hands and safely release your energy. You begin to connect again. You start to feel a little more pep in your step. You connect to your friend and yourself through these interactions. You are now in the ventral vagus system.

Sometimes it does not complete in this straightforward manner, and we become stuck in one or two parts of the system for extended periods. When we are in the dorsal vagal system for an extended period of time, this is known as depression. When we are in the sympathetic nervous system for long periods of time, we may refer to this as anxiety. Sometimes we become stuck between the two and fluctuate between dorsal and sympathetic, rarely feeling the ventral vagal. Our body has never completed its cycle and does not feel safe.

Critics of the polyvagal theory say that it is oversimplified and lacks scientific evidence. Scientific articles cite questions around the concept of three separate systems that do not communicate, and some oppose the theory, saying that the systems must communicate with each other and state that we are sometimes in multiple states at once. Critics report that heart rate discrepancies can be due to many biological factors and are not just managed by the nervous system. Critics also question whether mammals transitioned from reptiles in the evolutionary model or if there was a split in the evolutionary pattern. If this were true, it would create some questions about the theory (Grossman, 2023).

Our body systems and reactions are very complex, and it is challenging to prove them. The complex system of our body does not always make sense, leaving even the most prestigious scientists trying to figure it out. The polyvagal theory may oversimplify our reactions; however, sometimes, simple language allows us to understand the concepts in a way that we can use in our day-to-day lives.

I have decided to notice reactions as safety responses and have decided that other scientists can figure out why it happens. Whether there are separate systems is less important to me than the act of noticing why our body responds to specific phenomena and how we spontaneously respond. However, the concept of being more aware of how our body reacts and what it may be communicating is essential for growing resilience. It is a type of exposure exercise that allows our emotions to exist with purpose and efficiency. We can notice when we want to move as little as possible or when we want to get the heck out of the room. We can also see that our body is reacting to a safety response. At the same time, our mind knows we are safe. Recognizing these responses starts to build a superpower that eventually grows into resilience. The polyvagal theory provides clear language for discussing a complex natural bodily reaction straightforwardly. Due to its clarity, it can be beneficial to some as they start to notice their body reactions. Even as theory is still evolving, the language can still be helpful.

NATURAL REACTIONS

As I read neurological studies about the nervous system, I have become fascinated by our reactions on a deeper level. I notice how my body system responds, my client's body systems respond, and how people respond in day-to-day life. If you slow down and see your natural reactions throughout the day, you may find that they are similar to those of our ancestors trying to keep themselves safe from predators and natural threats.

Let's focus on the part of our evolution where we hunted and gathered berries for our nourishment. Let's pretend you are out collecting food for your family. You spot a saber-tooth tiger coming for you, and without even thinking, you run in the opposite direction and find a cave to sit in. You sit in that cave, shaking, hoping it did not see you go in. You may stare off into space, staying extremely still. Your breath is likely very slow and shallow, and your heart rate slows. At some point, your body naturally decides it must be safe, and you start to move again. You slowly realize you are still in the cave and move your limbs. Eventually, you step out of the cave in a daze. You figure out where you are and stumble back to your village. Your community asks, "What the hell happened to you?" and you tell the story. Everyone celebrates that you are alive, and the next day, you go back out to gather food. You are a little more cautious after your incident the previous day, but still able to function and know you are safe.

Let's rewrite this. This time, you turn around while gathering food, and a saber-tooth tiger is standing right beside you, ready to eat you. You faint, your heart slows to a very slow rate, and you are motionless. The tiger sniffs you and stands over you for some time, then decides you are deceased, sick, or not a nutritious meal. It moves on with its day. Eventually, you come back to reality, your body twitches and shakes, and you feel scared. You sit there for a bit, gathering your surroundings, and eventually realize you are safe.

What is the difference between these reactions and our current stress? We are no longer running from saber-tooth tigers. Our world is generally much safer than it once was. We get our food from the grocery store, and we have few, if any, natural predators. Most of us have a way to stay protected from the elements. Why do we respond in similar ways when our world is generally safe? The saber-tooth tiger is now perceptions of others, emotions we have deemed as unsafe, and thoughts that tear us down. We do not complete the emotion as I discussed above when we find safety, but rather override it, powering through so we can get to the next step. Our body doesn't have time to process the event and find safety; here we are stuck in the reaction loop, a response to danger. Will the things listed above kill us? Not immediately (there is an argument about long-term effects of stress that will indeed affect our health, but this is not what we are talking about in this moment). A mistake, a reaction from others, a thought, an emotion, all become a saber-tooth tiger about to kill us, but this time they won't kill us—they just feel like it. This is not a cognitive response. Our brain often knows we are safe. The physiological response, which does not always make logical sense, takes precedence over everyday logic. Theories around these spontaneous reactions to stimuli infer that, based on past experiences, the body system creates a response to things that may be unsafe in the future. The decision-making and conscious part of the brain has very little role in this (Šimić et al., 2021). I wonder if this is why some therapies are difficult to follow through with. When push comes to shove, our body will go to the default mode of safety, creating a variety of emotions along the way.

Our reactions to events, thoughts, and emotions are extremely complicated physiologically. When I begin explaining this concept, people get lost in their thoughts, wondering what each feeling means. For instance, if I get anxious, what am I nervous about? However, after many years of avoiding, we sometimes push the layers so far back that we cannot access them. This means that we are reacting to things without actually knowing what we are responding to. No matter how much we try to find the answer to why we just can't. We either come up with a reason for our anxiety (it must be XYZ) or we feel more lost, not understanding where it comes from. If we are at a restaurant and someone walks by who reminds us of our x significant other, who makes us very anxious, we become anxious again. Our body may decide that all restaurants are unsafe, and we don't even understand why. It may happen so quickly that we do not even notice that the connection was made. You start to wonder, "What makes restaurants unsafe and decide it must be the loud noise." You now avoid all places with loud noise. We can get lost in our thoughts very quickly, but when we are referring to stress responses, thoughts are not very helpful and can actually get in the way. I can tell you thoughts will come no matter what you are concentrating on. We spend enough time noticing thoughts. The ruminating loop often runs the show of our lives. Noticing physiology switches it up and creates space for things that don't make sense to our conscious thought. I am not saying thoughts are not important; they are very important, but they can just overshadow the other stuff if that is all we are concentrating on.

I am not naive enough to believe that no danger exists in our current world. We still need our nervous system for physical survival. In fact, large amounts of physical danger where we never find safety can also affect our nervous system in very real and significant ways. Examples of this would be lifetime family abuse, recurring natural disasters, and abusive relationships. I am grateful for our nervous system responses. They have kept us alive, and they continue to do so. When I step back, I see how shutting down is safer than being angry and scared in specific settings. I know "blending into the wallpaper" and not being seen can be much safer in certain situations when getting seen means getting in trouble. Our symptoms are not due to the nervous system response in itself; they often come from the mistrust of our nervous system reaction, creating a lack of safety in the response itself. This can be several layers deep. You see how it can get complicated quickly if we spend too much time trying to figure out every detail. Our system is remarkably intelligent when we allow it to function without getting in its way. It is just impossible to do this when we also have layers of stuff making it complicated. While you go through the process of finding safety within your reactions, you will find that your brain naturally knows whether it can allow for the frontal cortex to work and you can move out of your nervous system, or if you really need it. Your body will not relax the nervous system when you need it. I trust this because I have seen it time and time again. You do not have to trust this yet; it can be difficult to trust a body that has made you emotionally uncomfortable up to this point.

What does this look like in veterinary work? Your saber-tooth tigers have expanded. Your school was likely tough, and sometimes it felt like you would never graduate. It had high levels of stress that you may not have managed, more than turning on your grit and getting through it. This was likely necessary for you in the moment, but did you ever sit down and recognize that you are no longer in it? Many people jump straight from graduation to looking for or starting their first job. Entry-level positions have a lack of safety of their own. The pay, long hours, environments outside of your value system, and imposter syndrome of a new position can be very challenging. Did you ever find safety from this stress? Now you have been in the field longer. How much do you recognize your natural reactions to everyday things? The scared animal who is difficult because they do not trust you and try to protect themselves; the handler who is yelling at you, and you greatly disagree with their position; the young animal who has an illness that cannot be healed; that the handler who cannot afford to treat their pet; signs of animal abuse and neglect; and the expectations from yourself, your colleagues, and your handlers which are impossible to meet—all of these are your saber-tooth tigers. How much do you allow the emotion to complete themselves, and how much do you power through, never telling your body you are actually safe?

WINDOW OF TOLERANCE

Dan Siegel (1999) introduced to the therapy world the concept of a Window of Tolerance. This refers to the space in which people can feel an emotion, both comfortable and uncomfortable, and process it in the way that the body intends. When we feel our emotions within a space that it can process, we react to a known danger or threat, and our body finds safety and learns from the event (Hershler et al., 2021). As you can see in Figure 10.2, when we are in danger, our body first perceives the threat. It hears, sees, or senses danger in some way. After mobilizing in a way that the body feels safe, the system eventually realizes that it is safe from the interactions. The reactions turn down, and the emotion is complete, allowing us to return to life knowing we are safe.

We assume that processing for an event in your life takes about 8 weeks to process naturally. However, when our body is out of our window, it becomes more complicated, creating layers of emotions and reactions, making it difficult to process. The body begins to struggle with seeing and perceiving safety, creating safety responses that are no longer necessary. We now respond to the world as if everything is unsafe, creating unjustified reactions such as prolonged anxiety, ruminating thoughts, and feelings of disconnection and shutdown. We begin to avoid our emotions. We do not believe we should be angry, sad, guilty, etc. When we avoid the emotion, we communicate to our body system that we must be avoiding it because the emotion itself is unsafe. The emotion

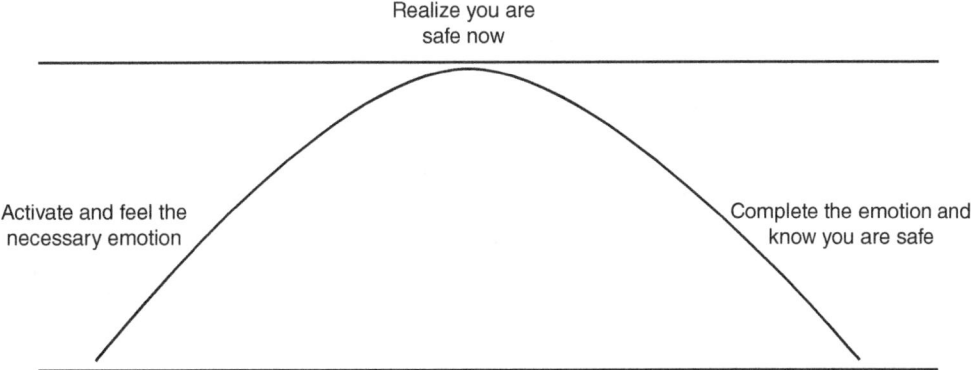

FIGURE 10.2   This image shows the bell curve of how an emotion presents itself and processing in a safe environment. When safety is not established, it is common for emotions to become stuck in one of these processes.

itself (which is a natural response and not inherently bad) has become the "bad guy." This makes it more challenging to return to our window of tolerance.

When we are hyperaroused and out of our window of tolerance, we often feel frantic, anxious, and experience ruminating thoughts, become hypervigilant, irritable, or feel like we want to run away or fight often. The saber-tooth tiger is perpetually in the corner of the room, and our brain is constantly trying to stay safe. Some refer to this as a fight or flight response; however, it is often more complicated than just fight or flight. Some emotions and reactions may not fit into those descriptions and still present themselves when we are hyperaroused.

When we are hypoaroused, we tend to have slower movement, a lack of motivation, difficulty concentrating, or depression. The saber-tooth tiger is constantly on top of us, and our bodies are trying to avoid the inevitable pain. Some refer to this as a freeze response; however, similar to the hyperarousal, there are reactions that people have in this state that do not fit that description.

You can see in Figure 10.3, that when we are in the window of tolerance, our body can complete the emotions; however, when we are hyperaroused or hypoaroused, we jump out of the window, struggling to find safety. Even though this picture does not depict it, we can go between

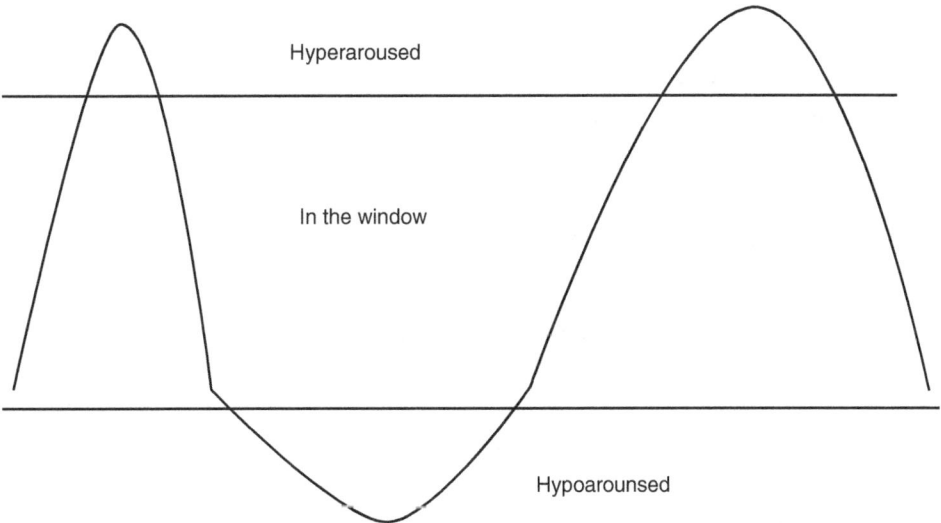

FIGURE 10.3   Window of tolerance. This figure shows the window of tolerance as well as hyper and hyperarousal.

hyperaroused and hypoaroused without going through our window. Imagine you can fold this picture into a tube shape. One may flow between hyperarousel and hypoarousel, or could go from either one into the window of tolerance.

There are several ways to re-enter our window of tolerance. Remember what I said about how the frontal cortex and the amygdala cannot work in the same capacity at the same time? By using your frontal cortex, you can remind yourself that you are safe. Here are some ways in which you can use your frontal cortex to remind yourself that you are safe. The struggle arises when you perform these tasks frantically, outside of your window of tolerance, rendering them ineffective. If you practice them as a way of just noticing and seeing, it takes the pressure off, and they are more likely to work. Notice that in each of these ideas, I end with a check-in with what you feel. If you do not periodically check in on how you feel about your current surroundings, even if it is uncomfortable, these strategies become avoidant rather than productive. If you avoid too much, the emotion can sneak up on you at a time when it is more difficult to manage. You will notice this exercise is not as step-by-step as some of the other ones are. I encourage you to try some of these out throughout your typical day. They are a great way to not only bring yourself back into your window, but also to check in to see if you are in or out of your window. When we are out of our window, we often do not notice until we check in. If you feel differently after doing a grounding exercise, you may have been out of your window.

EXERCISE 10.1 Grounding for getting back into the window

- Pick a color and notice all of the things in the room that are that color. How many shades of that color can you find? Check back in on your current situation.

- Notice if you hear any sounds in the room you have not noticed before. Spend some time being curious about sound. Check back in on your current situation.

- Use a strong-smelling lotion and pay attention to both the smell and how it feels on your hands. Check back in on your current situation.

- Find a coin and rub your hand around it, be curious about what you feel and where. Is it smooth or rough? Check back in on your current situation.

- Spend 3–5 minutes playing a phone game or a puzzle that challenges your thinking. Check back in on your current situation (Hendrickson et al., 2018).

- Try out some math equations. I like counting by 7, starting with 3, then trying it again backward. Check back in on your current situation (Greenwald, 2007).

- Throw a ball with a friend or by yourself. Throw it to different places so that you have to concentrate to catch it. Check back in on your current situation.

- Rub your thumb and index finger together. Become curious about where it is smooth and where it is rough. Can you feel your fingerprint? How is your nail different than the pad of your finger? Check back in on your current situation.

- Notice how you are sitting, standing, or lying in the room. Where does your body touch the furniture and ground? Where is there space? Provide as much detail as possible. Check back in on your current situation.

If you are significantly outside your window of tolerance, you may struggle to perform the skills above with success. In those cases, I encourage you to use the emergency skills below. You can trick your brain into being stressed about something else so that when you stop that event, your body knows you are sad. This allows you to go back to the original situation with more clarity. You will need to do some additional skills, as these skills are designed to be temporary relief, with the intention of bringing you closer to your window so that you can decide on effective next steps.

EXERCISE 10.2   Ice pack emergency skill

1. Hold two ice packs on your cheeks.

2. Hold your breath for 30 seconds.

3. After 30 seconds, remove the ice packs and return to your natural breathing.

4. Come back to the situation and see how you feel.

Your body believes you are diving underwater and sends all of its energy into helping you survive without drowning. When you begin breathing again, your body knows you are safe (Linehan, 2015).

EXERCISE 10.3   Exercise emergency skill

1. Select an exercise that you can perform without injuring yourself and is difficult enough that you become out of breath and need to concentrate on it.
   a. 100 jumping jacks
   b. A 1-minute wall sit
   c. 1-minute plank
   d. Standing on one foot for 3 minutes
   e. Circling your arms for 1 minute.

2. Do this exercise until you can think about nothing else except completing the exercise. If

you start shaking, that is perfectly okay. It actually can help with this process.

3. Allow your heart rate to increase and your breath to become strained.

4. Come back to the emotion.

Your body becomes preoccupied with surviving strenuous exercise, which mimics anxiety and stress. When you stop exercising, it calms itself, feeling as though it has survived the stress (Linehan, 2015).

EXERCISE 10.4   Inverted emergency skill

*This one is harder to do in public simply because people may think you are weird.

1. Find a way to invert yourself. Depending on your ability, you could choose between:

   a. Bending forward and touching your toes for a few minutes.
   b. Doing a handstand against the wall for a few minutes.
   c. Lying on a bed and letting your head hang over the side for a few minutes.

2. You may notice that the blood rushes to your head. Don't do this so long that you pass out,

just enough that your body feels off balance because it is upside down.

3. Sit back upright and let your body settle before getting up.

4. Come back to the situation and see how you feel.

Turning your body upside down sends the blood to the top of your head. This means the blood cannot flow to your extremities, where it thinks it should when you need to run or fight for something. When it flows back into your body, it flows into a more balanced state.

When we first start out exploring our window of tolerance, we may find that just being in the window is not safe. Our body has learned that a state of being grounded is unsafe. This shrinks our window, making it harder to get in. We can expand our window of tolerance by becoming aware of how our emotions present themselves in our bodies.

This can be highly challenging for some and easier for others. If any of these exercises bring up an increase in negative emotions or memories, please stop the exercise and contact a trained professional in your area.

When we notice how we feel the emotion in our body (even if we do not have a great name for the emotion itself), our body recognizes we are not dying from noticing and feeling the emotion, making the emotion itself safe. This is a form of exposure to the phobia we have toward our feelings and possible reactions. As you go through these steps, if there is a level that increases your anxiety, stop there and master that level before moving forward.

This is a process that can take practice to accomplish. I recommend practicing feeling emotions in small steps. Your window likely will not allow you to sit in your emotion for long periods of time or with great intensity. You can start by simply noticing the response in each level, saying hello to it, and then moving on with life, adding the next level at a later time. It can be shocking how much that brief moment can expand your awareness and resilience. If feeling your emotions in your body feels foreign and/or impossible, please be patient with yourself. This is one of those easier said than done skills. Powering through does not increase its effectiveness. In fact, it has the potential to make it ineffective.

You will notice that some of the ideas are reiterated from the Exercises in 10.1. The intention is different. In Exercise 10.1, you intend to ground. In Exercise 10.5, you intend to gain awareness of your emotions and how your body reacts to these emotions.

You will notice that we begin with awareness of our surroundings and progress to awareness of ourselves at a physical level, eventually developing internal awareness. I do not recommend jumping ahead. For certain levels can be very anxiety-provoking, popping us out of our window, making the exercises unproductive. You will notice that in all levels of the exercise, we will be using thought and curiosity about the world around us and ourselves. Both our thoughts and our emotions are important in this exercise so that both parts of the brain can work in a balanced way. The levels of awareness do not indicate if you are doing a "good or bad job," they are simply various levels of awareness for you to try out.

EXERCISE 10.5	Building layers of awareness to expand the window

Level 1: Awareness of your space

1. Start by looking around the room you are in.

2. Ask yourself, what do I see in this room that I have not noticed before? Focus on as much detail as possible.

3. Find one picture or object and begin to focus on the details of that. What is something you did not notice before? What is an interesting detail?

4. Take a moment and listen. Are there any noises that you can hear that you didn't notice before?

5. Pick a noise and see if you can notice any details in the noise.

6. Now, become curious about the smells in the room (good or bad). See if you can notice any smells you did not notice before.

7. After noticing the space, use these three senses to check in and see how you are in the space

now. Is it different or the same? *Remember, there is no correct answer.*

Level 2: Awareness of your body in the space

8. Notice how you are sitting, standing, or lying in this space?

9. Become curious about where your body hits the furniture or the floor and where there is space.

10. Become curious about how your body may feel different when it is touching something versus when it is not.

11. How are your feet? Where are they touching?

12. Where are your hands sitting? Do you notice anything about how they are resting on your skin or the area around you?

13. Notice how you feel after giving space to your senses and outside body in this space. Is it the same or different? *Remember, there is no correct answer.*

Level 3: Internal body awareness

14. Take a moment and notice your breath. You don't have to change it in this moment; just see it. It may change as you bring attention, just notice that.

15. Notice there is a natural pause in your breath at the top and at the bottom.

16. Notice where your breath naturally starts and stops in your body.

17. If you breath changes as you bring awareness to it, notice how it changes.

18. How do inhaling and exhaling feel different?

19. Are there any catches in your breath where breath is more difficult? Are the catches in the inhale, exhale, or both?

20. If you feel comfortable, explore what it feels like to breath a little longer and/or a little deeper.

21. Are there any different catches? How is this different, and how is it the same?

22. Notice if you feel different after becoming more aware of your breath or if you feel the same. *Remember, there are no right answers.*

Level 4: Becoming aware of emotions in the body

23. Do a scan of your body. For those who prefer a visualization, I like to picture a black light scanning my body, highlighting various areas I can be curious about.

24. Pick a part of your body that feels interesting to you. It can be significant or not.

25. Bring your awareness to the sensation. *Example: I feel a tightness in my chest.*

26. Ask yourself, does it have a color, a shape, or a temperature?

27. How deep or shallow is the sensation?

28. As you bring attention, does it move or change? If it does, just follow it.

29. What spontaneous thoughts (if any) come up as you notice the sensation?

30. Become curious about this sensation for as long as you can tolerate.

EMOTIONS AS FRIEND, NOT FOE

"Emotions are a noun, not a verb". This is a phrase I use multiple times a day. People ask, "What does it mean?"

We often describe our responses to our emotions as our emotions. We say, "I got angry," instead of "I feel angry." This communicates that the only way to be angry is to yell at everyone, stomp your feet, and act aggressively. The only way to be sad is to cry in the corner, and the only way to be anxious is to be a jittery mess worried about everything around you. What if you can be angry, notice your desire to punch the next person you see, say hi to the anger, and decide what to do with it? Sounds a little magical, doesn't it? What if you can notice your anxiety, label it as a tight chest and difficulty breathing, and allow it to work itself out without getting worse and starting to spiral? Think about how much control you may have over your life. The phrase I use, "Emotions are a noun, not a verb," refers to the idea that the emotion is not how you act, so it cannot be a verb. It also does not describe who you are, and it cannot be an adjective. Instead, it is a thing, making it a noun.

Not only are emotions a thing, but they are a thing with a purpose. Each of our emotions as an individual purpose that has kept us alive for many years. You can see these in the chart (Figure 10.4). Please note that the chart is very simple compared to our extraordinarily complicated emotions. You may also see that some of the boxes overlap. Before understanding the complexity of emotions and reactions, a primary start is to notice it in simple terms, knowing it might not make sense quite yet. Easier said than done, I know, but just try it.

Going deeper into Figure 10.4, I want to discuss how these emotions have served us through the years. Some of these emotions we consider to be "bad." Sometimes we even hate the emotion, creating a complex system of avoidance. Think about it in the context of the herd mentality. If we did not have grief, anger, or guilt, how could we survive as a community? Certain cultures see tears as a weakness. However, tears are a very important part of how humans communicate emotions to each other. When we see someone cry, we have a desire to help them and connect with them. Sadness has a desire to isolate because it is so painful that it does not feel worth it to connect; however, connection is essential to our vitality. Tears allow us to communicate through the deepest of pain. The act of crying also involves body movement and facial expressions that create a relief from the emotion that we feel (Gračanin, Bylsma and Vingerhoets, 2014; Sznycer, Gračanin and Lieberman, 2025).

Anger is designed to protect our land from other tribes. If we did not defend our physical boundaries, we would be taken over by other animals or other traditions. Sometimes the boundary crossed is emotions, while other times it is physical. It communicates to us that we should protect ourselves and makes us scary enough that the threat wants to go away. Guilt is designed to tell us that we did something outside of our values and morals, or the values and morals within the system. If we did not have guilt, people within the tribal community would begin to harm each other, thus putting the tribe in danger. Worry is designed to help us prepare for the future. We actually need it to be able to say what we will do and respond appropriately to a crisis situation. Since our logic part of the brain works less during dangerous situations, planning ahead allows space to build muscle memory, making it more likely we will respond appropriately when needed. It is designed to be a brief emotion designed for preparation. Happiness is needed to balance all of the difficult emotions and create lasting connections with ourselves and others. It communicates to us that we are nurturing ourselves and our community. We feel happiness, joy, and connection when we are feeling safe.

Our emotions are very complicated. Sometimes they appear when they are not needed. *For example, I feel guilty for saying no to a request even though I know it is important and others are not offended.* Sometimes they have multiple layers because the emotion itself triggers additional emotions. *For example, we have been told sadness is a weakness, so now we have guilt that we are sad. We become aware of this and become angry because we feel guilty about our sadness.* Sometimes we know exactly what emotion we are feeling in a given moment, and it appears clearly and recognizably, like this chart. Sometimes we feel multiple emotions at one time, or we feel the emotion more in our body than our mind, so it makes less sense. There are also a million different names for emotions that allow us to get very specific about each. I find it easiest to start noticing the bigger, simpler names of emotions and label them when possible, instead of trying to label each and every moment of every day with the most detailed word possible. With the knowledge of the purpose of each emotion, we can become aware of them, whether they are needed in the moment or not.

Emotion	What it feels like	What is its purpose
Sad	• Desire to isolate • Tearful • Feeling like it will never be better • Slow movement	• Connect to others • A need for support from others • An ability to connect to others when they are sad
Angry	• Irritability • A desire to leave, stomp, or hit • Energy in the body • Tight muscles • A desire to growl (Vocal sigh)	• Communicates that someone crossed a boundary or value • Protection of yourself and those you love
Anxious/Scared	• A pull back motion • A desire to get out or step away • A tight chest • A jitteriness or a desire to move • Shallow quick breath • Thinking about the future almost all of the time • Racing thoughts about you or your loved ones being in danger	• To get us out of an unsafe situation that could put us in danger
Guilty	• Ruminating thoughts about having done something wrong • Constant wish you could go back in time • A desire to hide	• Communicates that you are acting outside of your value system or the values of society
Disgust	• Nauseous feeling • A desire to get away from something • Difficult being around whatever you may be disgusted by	• Protection from poisoning
Joy/happiness	• Connection to yourself, others, and your environment • Smiling • Desire to keep doing fun things	• Connection to yourself, others, and your environment • This is nurturing, you should keep doing it.

FIGURE 10.4 Purpose of emotions. Emotions are listed in the first column, the way the emotion is seen is in the second column, and the purpose of emotions is in the third column. This chart can be used to understand emotions in a deeper way and in order to determine when emotions are justified or unjustified.

So, why do you feel guilty when you set a boundary you know you need to set, or feel angry that someone wore a pink shirt today? Logic and emotion begin to disconnect when emotions are not justified. The body is responding to old messages from our community, avoidance of emotions or situations or messages we receive throughout our lives about the way things should be. Some of these messages are presented obviously (parents saying you should not cry because it is weak) or less obviously (people ignoring you when you cry or only listening when you yell). Sometimes we know exactly where this disconnect came from; sometimes we do not. Our job is to become aware of our emotions as they happen so that we can decide if they are justified or not. As we do this, we gain the ability to listen to the emotion or do the opposite since it is not needed in that situation. How we developed unjustified emotions is less important than the fact that they exist.

I can't tell you how many times someone has come into therapy to get rid of an emotion. Unfortunately, getting rid of an emotion is getting rid of both the justified adaptive response and the unjustified maladaptive response. We need these emotions, or we might stand too close to tall ledges or walk into a dark cave with an angry critter inside. While we cannot get rid of emotions, we can slow them down by noticing them and our bodily reactions, so that we have more control over deciding what to do with them. Eventually, we train our emotions to respond more rationally.

Think of emotions as if they are small children pulling on your pants legs while you talk with other adults. Sometimes it does not make sense to respond to them immediately. You may say, "I am having an adult conversation one moment." If you do not say anything at all, they get more annoying and naughtier. If you pause when you have a moment and ask what they need, they often communicate a need you can say yes or no to. Sometimes they say "I forgot," "I want a Popsicle," or "oh, nothing," and run off. They simply needed to be seen. If we say we will answer them in a moment and forget to answer them, they will calm down for a moment, but will become loud and naughty again when time has passed. Done multiple times, they will no longer calm when you say "Wait a moment," because they do not believe you will actually listen. In the same way, our emotions will tug on us and annoy us, getting louder and naughtier the more we ignore them. If we stop for a moment and ask what they need, they may communicate something important, or turn down their intensity. You do not have to stop every moment, as you may be busy, distracted, or talking to other adults, but making time to check in on them for moments at a time can give them more space to communicate what you need effectively.

AVOIDANCE

Humans really like to avoid uncomfortable things. We have labeled many reactions and emotions as useless and unsafe. There are many generations of messages communicating what is safe and unsafe, even if it doesn't apply in our world today. It makes sense to avoid discomfort sometimes. It would be difficult to effectively practice veterinary medicine if you were worried about the fight you had with your significant other earlier in the day. We need to function in the many roles we hold in our world. I need to do my job, be a parent, a friend, a son/daughter/child (etc.). The problem is that when we avoid our emotions for long periods of time and never come back to them, we start to communicate that they are dangerous. When we communicate that they are dangerous, every time we feel the emotion, we then feel fear or anxiety around the emotion itself. Now it becomes a dangerous emotion, and our system becomes endlessly complicated. It becomes harder for us to enter into our window of tolerance because the saber-tooth tiger our body is convinced will kill us is extremely complicated. Animotophobia is the fear of emotions. I would be willing to say a large percentage of people who seek treatment from me have some level of animotophobia. I can honestly say that I have some below-the-surface animotophobia I wasn't even aware of until I accidentally treated it in my late 20s.

When we create a habit of avoiding emotions, we also avoid all things that may cause our emotions. This is why we may begin to have an urge to avoid work, certain people, or situations where we have felt the emotion before (even if that situation was not directly related to the emotion). As we avoid or have the urge to avoid these places, people, and situations, we start to communicate to our body system that all places are unsafe. Our emotions become bigger, and we develop a broader range of triggers to that emotion.

As you start to practice awareness instead of avoidance, your body will begin to recognize that your world is safer than it once thought. It is a brief exposure to the situation, emotion, or both. When we have the willingness to be uncomfortable for a moment at a time, things naturally slow down. This can be an extensive process for some. I do not recommend doing this in significant ways and exposing yourself to the emotions in the most extreme way possible. After avoiding emotions and situations for many years, it will likely be challenging to begin noticing them again. Trying to notice all the emotions all the time in their greatest intensity can be a recipe for jumping out of your window, making the awareness more difficult or impossible. Allow yourself to take small steps. Start with an emotion that you avoid and can tolerate. If you experience uncomfortable emotions for long periods of time without professional help, you may become overwhelmed and potentially exacerbate the issue. Instead, I recommend exposing yourself and exploring this in brief, tolerable moments.

FOOD FOR THOUGHT JOURNAL TOPIC:

1. Review a typical Day. How does your nervous system react on a given day (both effective and ineffective)?

2. What are the signs that you are out of your window of tolerance and acting on your emotions?

REFERENCES

Gračanin, A., Bylsma, L. M. and Vingerhoets, A. J. (2014). 'Is crying a self-soothing behavior?', *Frontiers in Psychology*, 5, p. 502.

Greenwald, R. (2007). *EMDR Within a Phase Model of Trauma-Informed Treatment.* New York: Haworth Press.

Grossman, P. (2023). 'Fundamental challenges and likely refutations of the five basic premises of the polyvagal theory', *Biological Psychology*, 180, 108589.

Hendrickson, K. L., Rasmussen, R. C., Yi, R. J. and Levin, M. E. (2018). 'Effects of Mindful Eating Training on Delay and Probability Discounting', *Behaviour Research and Therapy*, 109, pp. 31–38.

Hershler, A., Hughes, L., Nguyen, P. and Wall, S. (2021) *Looking at Trauma: A tool Kit for Clinicians.* Pennsylvania: Penn State University Press.

Linehan, M. M. (2015). *DBT® Skills Training Handouts and Worksheets* (2nd ed.). New York: The Guilford Press.

O'Connor, M.-F. (2022). *The Grieving Brain.* Pinhurst, NC: O'Connor Production Inc.

Porges, S. (2023). *Polyvagal theory: Summary, premises & current status.* Polyvagal Institute, 8e115bf8 f82f01065b41dc85e7698fd4f99818.pdf

Porges, S. W. (2022). '*Polyvagal theory: A science of safety*', *Frontiers in Integrative Neuroscience*, 16, 871227.

Siegel, D. J. (1999). *The Developing Mind: Toward a Neurobiology of Interpersonal Experience.* New York: Guilford Press.

Šimić, G. *et al.* (2021). 'Understanding emotions: Origins and roles of the amygdala', *Biomolecules*, 11(6), p. 823. https://doi.org/10.3390/biom11060823.

Sznycer, D., Gračanin, A. and Lieberman, D. (2025). 'Emotional tears: What they are and how they work', *Evolution and Human Behavior*, 46(1), 106652.

CHAPTER 11

Well-Being from a Nervous System Perspective: Tying It All Together

If you are sick of being irritable, followed by guilt about this irritability, or if you are hard on yourself for not following through with the tasks and goals you set out to do, good news, you don't have to be mad at yourself anymore. You can recognize that this is part of your nervous system, trying to keep you safe. It is just a little bit confused about what is safe and what is not safe. Either overtly or covertly, a reaction or a person or a group of people has communicated to you that something is unsafe, and your body has interpreted it. That does not mean I expect you to go around being irritable and telling everyone it's okay because it is a physiological response. It simply means being curious about reactions in a different way. I am making it sound easy, and I am sure you will continue to be mad at yourself at times. I just want you to have access to alternative options.

We often go through life just letting reactions happen. We either feel guilty or weak because we cannot control them. We feel frustrated that they come up no matter how much work we have done to develop skills to avoid them. Sometimes, we even resort to blaming everyone else for making us react. If we slow down a half beat and recognize that these reactions are biological and designed for safety, we can gain some control over them and allow ourselves to have these reactions while also deciding what is truly dangerous (Bayes, Tavella and Parker, 2021; Mikołajewska *et al.*, 2022).

When we discuss work-related stress responses like burnout, compassion fatigue, and vicarious trauma, these are responses to the work itself becoming unsafe. Physiologically, we begin to respond to the job as if it were a predator about to eat us. There is a combination response where we want to run but feel stuck and frozen. Our body is scared that if we move too much, we might die, but we are so uncomfortable that we just want to leave, wanting nothing more than to crawl under a blanket and never get out. That sounds a lot like a cave to me. A place you can retreat and hide, moving very little so that the threat cannot attack. When brain imaging is done on people experiencing burnout and this is compared to a control group, differences are found in the amygdala and frontal cortex. These are also the safety parts of the brain.

COMPASSION FATIGUE FROM A NERVOUS SYSTEM PERSPECTIVE

Compassion fatigue is often caused by creating space for difficult situations in the past without the skills to manage it. You begin to feel compassion, and as you feel deep compassion, pain can sometimes follow. You hold both your own emotions and those of everyone you have come into contact with that day. You are too busy and skilled at avoidance, and you avoid the feelings that arise when you are compassionate about difficult situations. Because the pain has not been addressed and you shove it down, going about your day, your body believes that you are avoiding these emotions because they are unsafe. This creates a message that compassion is dangerous, over time, creating a disconnect from all things around you, sometimes even creating a disconnection to compassion for yourself.

BURNOUT FROM A NERVOUS SYSTEM PROSPECTION

Burnout happens when the job and/or career becomes unsafe. The body responds to the job as if it were a threat. There are countless reasons why a job may become unsafe, but here are just a few that may fit:

- The stress from the intensity of the job has not been addressed. Stress is not safe to the body, so it labels the job as a whole as unsafe.

- The job threatens a value of yours. This threatens something meaningful to the way you are or the way you believe the world should be.

- Emotional exhaustion has not been addressed, and the emotions that the job creates become unsafe, over time creating a message that the whole job or career is unsafe.

- Someone or something at work is very similar to something unsafe in the past, and the body system lumps them together.

- Time at work is interfering with other parts of your life, which create safety (enjoyment, family, friends, and other connections). Without balancing stress with fun, your body feels like your whole world is unsafe.

- Doing something wrong or being perceived as wrong is threatening to you and shows up daily in the job.

If none of these rings true for you and you are still burnt-out, don't worry. The reason for the feeling of threat is not as important as how we deal with it.

Because the job has become unsafe, and you are expected to be there most days of the week for many hours, it becomes a saber-tooth tiger waiting outside of the cave, relentlessly waiting for you to come out. If a saber-tooth tiger were sitting outside of your cave waiting for you to come out, you may eventually turn off your emotions because they feel too big or feel trapped. If the job is a saber-tooth tiger you are living beside each day, no wonder burnout is so exhausting. You start to move more slowly (body functions slow to avoid pain if you are attacked), the frontal cortex, or thinking part of the brain, is reacting less than the brain stem or safety part of the brain, creating a greater possibility for mistakes and slower thinking patterns. You want to run as far away from work as possible, meaning you may watch the clock, have to drag yourself into work each day, or have a desire to work as little as possible. I would want to run as far away from predators that were trying to eat me.

When brain imaging is done on people experiencing burnout and this is compared to a control group, differences are found in the amygdala and frontal cortex. These are also the safety parts of the brain.

VICARIOUS/SECONDARY TRAUMA FROM A NERVOUS SYSTEM PERSPECTIVE

For reasons we do not fully understand, sometimes things become stuck, creating symptoms of trauma. The theory that best fits this for me is the Adaptive informational processing (AIP) model (Shapiro, 2018). This model assumes that in a memory that processes thoroughly all parts of the brain are working to their fullest. I think of this as a toddler toy where each shape goes into its respective part. The five senses are each a shape that is assigned to a specific spot in the brain, allowing the brain to make sense of the event and find safety again. Sometimes, our brain gets confused and tries to fit the triangle into the circular space, making it difficult for the brain to complete the memory. The memory now floats around in the brain as if it is happening in the here and now, even though it is not. This creates confusion within the reactions as it is unclear if you are living the experience which was once unsafe or living in the safer world you live in now. Your system relives the experience as if it is happening right now. Your logic brain knows you are not, but your system believes that you are.

MORAL INJURY FROM A NERVOUS SYSTEM PERSPECTIVE

You have made a mistake that your body system has interpreted so far outside of your own personal value system that you label yourself as a bad person. You followed the orders of a clinic that runs things outside of your primary work values. You performed a procedure requested by a handler that you do not believe you should have. You were told to react to customers in a way you greatly disagree with; whatever the event that happened, you so greatly wish that you had responded differently that you now deem yourself a threat to your community. You feel like you could cause harm to others because, in your own mind, you are the saber-tooth tiger. You wish you could run away from yourself or fight yourself to protect your community. You may isolate or have desires to punish yourself, sometimes even having suicidal thoughts, due to these safety responses. You may carry large amounts of shame, believing you must be a bad person. You may or may not logically know that you are doing the best you can within the structure.

IMPOSTER SYNDROME

Entering a challenging career with multiple moving parts, like veterinary medicine, has an inevitable consequence of imposter syndrome. Feeling like you are not good enough, even when people are giving you positive feedback. The idea of judgment from others, not meeting expectations, and making mistakes can become detrimental to the mind. Sometimes, this is because you are scared that people may notice your flaws; sometimes it is simply fear that you are not good at this job you worked so hard to get into; and other times, it is fear that you will make a dire mistake. Whatever the reason for your imposter syndrome, it can be defined as a phobia of doing something wrong and not being good enough. The after effects include debilitating anxiety, indecisiveness, ruminating thoughts, and low self-esteem.

You may notice that telling yourself you are doing well or that imposter syndrome is normal does not give enough relief to manage the thoughts. Trying to push away the thoughts only makes them worse. The imposter syndrome is screaming so loud through the argument that the imposter syndrome or the argument becomes unsafe. Sometimes both feel unsafe, leading to a more trapped feeling.

DECISION-MAKING FATIGUE FROM A NERVOUS SYSTEM PERSPECTIVE

Ugh, the number of decisions you make in a given day in your field is exhausting. Many of these decisions are time-sensitive, high-intensity, and judged and scrutinized by colleagues, handlers, and yourself. Over time, these decisions have become so incredibly stressful that decision-making has become unsafe. There is so much fear that you will make the wrong decision that decision-making has become the predator about to eat you. When you are trying to decide on the best care, you become frozen or work very slowly. When someone asks you what you want for dinner, you become frozen, experience racing thoughts, or become highly anxious. The body has created a path in the brain that communicates all decisions as unsafe.

NEUROSIS FROM A NERVOUS SYSTEM PERSPECTIVE

Coping ahead is a skill. It allows us to manage anxiety by planning for the worst-case scenario. Neurosis simply takes a much-needed skill for survival and amplifies it to the point where it becomes less productive. The brain becomes scared it will miss something and not be prepared. It then develops this hypervigilance and need to notice and prepare for bad things constantly. Positive events become a danger because they distract from the ability to prepare. In addition, mistakes have become unsafe. People seeing you as incompetent is the bear in the room, and the body is responding in a way to avoid it. If you catch all of the tiny details, you will not make a mistake, which will avoid the feeling of incompetence. You strive for an impossible task, perfectionism. Each time you do not reach the impossible goal, you build more information that mistakes are not safe, exacerbating the symptoms.

A young girl I know was getting very anxious with sight words when she was learning to read. Someone taught her some breathing exercises to calm her thoughts and explained the concept of the sight words being "a bear." The body feels like the sight words are a threat, even though they will not kill you. For many months, she would take a deep breath and say, "It is not a bear." Maybe we need to be just as literal as this young child, reminding ourselves *deep breath in "it is not a bear"— Exhale. This allows our body to be comfortable with letting our guard down slowly and allowing small amounts of exposure to being more comfortable with emotions and their reactions within our body.

HERE ARE SOME ADDITIONAL SYMPTOMS AND HOW THEY RELATE TO THE NERVOUS SYSTEM PERSPECTIVE

Irritability: When a predator threatens us, we need to look bigger and meaner than it is to scare it away. Our body system becomes impulsively irritable with people around us to protect us from the possibility that they might be a threat. Sometimes irritability also comes from fear that you are not seen, which can feel unsafe to the body system as well. Everyone wants to feel important, and everyone wants to be respected for their hard work. It is important to feel part of the herd. If you are not seen, it becomes a threat to the necessity of your being part of the group (subconsciously, the logical mind knows you are important).

Cynicism: is your body's preparation for the worst. It constantly focuses on the negative, fearing you might miss something that could hurt you. Coping ahead and thinking about how to manage a difficult situation in the future is a practical skill; cynicism takes it a bit too far.

Racing thoughts: When we have racing thoughts, it is often because a perceived threat is close and our brain is trying to decide how to deal with it. If a predator were on the other side of the room, your brain would naturally race through several ways to stay safe. This is what the brain is doing with racing thoughts. Racing thoughts are often a sign that we are out of our window. It is proof that our thoughts cannot find safety, so they have to keep racing. Sometimes racing thoughts are your brain fearing you will forget important information that could keep you safe. It feels as though you need to keep thinking about it so you don't forget.

Difficulty concentrating: The safety part of our brain, which starts in the brain stem, and the problem-solving part of the brain in the frontal cortex cannot work at the same time. If a beast came into the room you are sitting in and someone beside you asked you what $2+2$ was, you would say "I don't care" (or more likely, throw out some expletives) and try to get safe. When our safety response is on, our frontal cortex moves slower creating brain fog and difficulty concentrating.

Worry: Your body is preparing for something. It has not found safety, so it holds the message that the world will never be safe. The safest thing to do is to prepare for the other shoe to drop. You must prepare for everything that could go wrong, because it inevitably will go wrong. We sometimes ruminate on worry because our brain is scared we will forget to worry and not be prepared.

Disconnection or numb: Our body does not want to feel physical pain, so it developed a mechanism that disconnects so that extreme pain cannot be felt. When our emotions become extremely painful, our body treats them as if they are physical pain and disconnects in the same way. If we disconnect from others, they cannot hurt us. If we disconnect from ourselves, we do not have to feel pain (physical or emotional). If we disconnect from our environment and/or nature, we do not have to acknowledge that we are present within it. The disconnection response is a natural defense mechanism where our body system gets tired of responding to the stress, so it simply turns off the source of the stress, which is the connection. This sounds great in theory, but it can be very uncomfortable when one also disconnects from joy, love, and passion. When we are disconnected from ourselves and others, it becomes increasingly difficult to empathize with those around us, leading to compassion fatigue.

Snappiness: When you are in a dangerous situation, you must act quickly. If your body is ready and treats each situation as if it were a dangerous situation, it will act swiftly and aggressively to "get stuff done." Yes, people need to act quickly in a veterinary office; however, the snappiness is less needed and more impulsive. The difficult addition to snappiness is that it trickles down, because as you are snappy at others, they feel unsafe, and they respond to the next person with snappiness, and the cycle begins and continues.

Slow moving: When other defenses do not work, our body gives up and begins to respond from a more freeze state. If an animal in the wild is immobile, other animals assume it is diseased and will often pass by it, looking for a healthier meal. The body system communicates that if you move quickly, you will draw attention to yourself and thus become a target for predators. Without any conscious thought, our body begins to move slowly, no matter how hard we wish it were moving faster. It is afraid we will get eaten if we move too fast.

Stuck feeling: When your body is recognizing all of the negatives in the world, as it does with intense stress, it begins to feel stuck. It feels as though there is no way out of the difficult situation. The stuck feeling is part of the freeze response, a feeling as though nothing will work to make things easier. Sometimes it is a combination of the fight/flight defense mechanism and freeze response, and our body system cannot decide which one makes sense, making us feel stuck.

Chronic stress/overwhelm: The nervous system is not designed to feel unsafe all of the time. It is designed to have moments of reaction and moments of safety. When we never relieve ourselves from stress, the body responds to every situation as if it is dangerous, sending constant chemicals throughout the body in response to the stress. We fluctuate between fight, flight, and freeze, and sometimes all three, or some combination of them, without any logical rhyme or reason.

Perfectionism: the need to be perfect stems from a wide variety of safety responses. Your body system has developed a belief that if you make a mistake, you will die. This stems from the importance of doing the right thing or emphasizing the quality of care. Quality of care is essential in the field, and I do not believe this should change. It is simply important for veterinarians to understand where perfectionism comes from. People hear stories about other veterinarians who make a mistake and get professionally destroyed by the action, or who become so distressed that they cannot perform in the same way. They fear that a mistake will happen in the same way, which creates extreme worry and anxiety, to the point of overthinking or freezing.

REFERENCES

Bayes, A., Tavella, G. and Parker, G. (2021). 'The biology of burnout: Causes and consequences', *The World Journal of Biological Psychiatry*, 22(9), pp. 686–698.

Mikołajewska, E. *et al.* (2022). 'From neuroimaging to computational modeling of burnout: The traditional versus the fuzzy approach—A review', *Applied Sciences*, 12(22), p. 11524.

Shapiro, F. (2018). *Eye Movement Desensitization and Reprocessing (EMDR) Therapy: Basic Principles, Protocols, and Procedures* (3rd ed.). New York: Guilford Press.

CHAPTER 12

Moving from Reaction to Settled

The first step in responding to reactions from a nervous system perspective is to understand your responses from a nervous system perspective. Noticing your body working toward safety, even when it is annoying, slows the process down slightly so that you have more room to address it. Once you decide how your system is responding based on a safety response, you can begin to build safety in your body.

EXERCISE 12.1 Exercise for a response that is more shut down, creating movement

1. Rub your hands together to create friction

2. Notice what your hands feel like as they generate heat through the movement

3. Rub your arms as if you are getting something gross off of them

4. Rub your face as if you are getting something gross off of it

5. Check in. How do you feel now?

Why this works: When you are beginning to feel shut down, small movements communicate to your body that you are safe. In addition, when you do not die from these small movements, your system is reassured. Shut down would include times you are moving more slowly, feel tired for no reason, have difficulty concentrating, or want to crawl into a hole. Your body believes that if you move too much, you will die. The predator is standing directly over you, about to eat you, and you need to play dead (Dana, 2020).

EXERCISE 12.2 Exercise for a response that is more shut down, drink warm liquid

1. Make a warm liquid, preferably something not caffeinated if caffeine creates anxiety for you.

2. Feel what the warm cup feels like on your hands.

3. Notice what it feels like to smell the drink and feel the heat on your face.

4. Drink warm liquid

5. Notice what it feels like as you swallow the drink and it enters your system

Why this works: When the body starts to shut down, it often feels colder. The blood flow is slower. When you drink warm liquid, it creates a faster blood flow which tells the body it must be safe.

EXERCISE 12.3   Exercise for a response that is more shut down, Math

1. Make up some simple math problems and solve them. Something like $2 + 2 = 4$, $4 + 4 = 8$, and $8 + 8 = 16$, and see how far you can go.

2. Move to a cognitive task for work that requires math or emotionless problem-solving.

Why this works: When your brain is responding to a safety response, your frontal cortex (thinking part of your brain) is working less than your amygdala (safety response). Your body has to decide which one it wants to use. Unless you are actually in danger, it will choose the safest option (Gregory, 2012).

EXERCISE 12.4   Exercise for a response that is more activated

These exercises are designed for times when you feel more activated. Times when you have racing thoughts, intense anxiety or worry, or want to run from the building as fast as you can (I will go over irritability separately, but these can also work for that).

1. Pick an exercise you can do for a minute (or maybe a minute and a half if you exercise hard, often). Ideas: wall sit, jumping jacks, run in place, or stomping around.

2. Do this exercise to the best of your ability.

3. Check in on the experience that activated you. Sometimes this is a broad ("I hate my job"),

sometimes it is more specific ("That visit sucked"). The discomfort likely has not gone away, but the hope is that it turns down enough that you can go about your day and/or see it more clearly.

Why this works: If we can do something that distracts us entirely to a point that we have no choice but to distract, we can successfully reset the loop created in the nervous system. In addition to this, the movement can communicate to your body that you effectively ran away from the predator (Dana, 2020).

EXERCISE 12.5   Exercise for a response that is more activated Tetris

1. Play Tetris for 1–2 minutes. You can find Tetris on many smartphones, computers, and video game consoles.

2. Was it too easy? Move to whatever level is challenging enough to create some stress.

Why does this work? There are three studies (Butler *et al.*, 2020; Holmes *et al.*, 2009; Iyadurai *et al.*, 2017; Hagenaars *et al.*, 2017) that prove that Tetris can effectively treat trauma and intense stress.

Why Tetris: The stress of the game relocates the stress into something that completes itself. If you lose at a game of Tetris, you do not die. If you lose in a fight with a predator, well, you're not playing Tetris anytime soon. In addition, there are

bilateral movements within the game of Tetris. One must quickly scan the whole screen to see where there are openings for the piece. When a person is appropriately processing a stressful situation, they utilize both sides of the brain, and it is not uncommon for the brain to make micro movements back and forth. The back and-forth movements elicit processing. Lastly, it also uses your frontal cortex. This is the decision-making part of the brain, which cannot run at the same time as the amygdala, the danger response part of the brain. One has to let go of the other, and the one that actually fits the facts of the situation wins. This means that if you are not actually in danger, the frontal cortex takes over, and you feel safer.

EXERCISE 12.6 Exercise for a response that is more activated: Cold liquid

1. Make an icy nonalcoholic drink. Water works best with this.

2. Notice how the cup feels in your hands.

3. Drink the cold liquid. Notice what it is like.

Avoiding alcohol and caffeine is highly recommended.

   Why this works: When your body is in an activated response, it is likely to be warmer. The blood flow is faster and most likely in your limbs more than your central body, as it is preparing to run away or fight or do whatever it needs to do to get away from the predator that is just far enough away that you can be safe. When you drink cold liquid, it naturally cools the body, telling it that it is safer than it once thought. In addition, dehydration can create a feeling of anxiety. Drinking water can hydrate you if it is related to your symptoms (Dana, 2020).

EXERCISE 12.7 Basic nervous system reset: Stanley Rosenberg's "The Basic Exercise"

This exercise is beneficial for some, as they reset their nervous system, and less helpful for others. Try it out and see how it works for you.

1. Place your hands on the back of your head so that your thumbs touch the part of the neck where the head and neck connect.

2. Turn your head to look around the room. Move your head right to left and left to right a few times.

3. Pause looking straight ahead.

4. Allow your eyes to wander to the right side as far as they can go while your head stays straight.

5. Let them rest here until you yawn, belch, your breath changes, or for a few moments.

6. Move your eyes to the left side with your head staying straight.

7. Let your eyes rest here until you yawn, belch, your breath changes, or for a few moments.

8. Come to the middle

9. Move your head from side to side, looking around the room, and see if your range of motion shifted.

10. Check in on your nervous system. How are you feeling?

You can stop here or continue.

11. Move your head so that your right ear rests on your right shoulder or close to it. You do not have to stretch too much, just whatever is comfortable.

12. Allow your left ear to move to the left shoulder.

13. Move back to the right ear, facing the right shoulder. Allow your eye to drift to the corner as if it is trying to look at your right shoulder. Sit here until you belch, yawn, or your breath changes, or for a few moments.

14. Move so that your left ear faces your left shoulder. Allow your eye to drift to the corner as if you are looking at your left shoulder. Sit here until you belch, yawn, your breath changes, or for a few moments.

15. Return to the center and check in to see if anything has changed (Rosenberg, 2017).

Why this works: When your body perceives danger, it tends to focus with tunnel vision. By looking around the room and moving your eyes into peripheral vision, you communicate to your nervous system that you are in a safe environment, as you are not fixating on a single point with tunnel vision.

EXERCISE 12.8 Grounding with a Tennis Ball

Sometimes we have no idea whether we are above our window or below it; we simply feel disoriented. It may be hard to tell what you are thinking or if you are thinking anything at all. Perhaps you are struggling to understand what you are reading or what people are saying. This is a great way to ground yourself when you are not sure what else to do.

1. Grab a Tennis Ball, take off your shoes, and stand beside the tennis ball.

2. Pick a foot to start with and roll the ball along the bottom of your foot.

3. Find a place near the pad of your foot (near your toes) and step down on the ball as you inhale. Release as you exhale.

4. Repeat in this same spot three times.

5. Roll the ball around again. Find a place in the Arch of your foot (In the middle) and press down as you inhale and release as you exhale.

6. Repeat this three times on this spot.

7. Roll the ball around your foot again, stopping somewhere on your heel. As you inhale, press down on the spot as you exhale, release.

8. Do this three times.

9. Set the ball aside and see if you feel different on the floor.

10. Move to the other foot and repeat steps 2–8 with the other foot.

11. Take a moment to notice if you feel any different after completing this exercise.

EXAMPLE OF THE NERVOUS SYSTEM AND IMPOSTER SYNDROME

First, you notice your thoughts or reactions. You may notice thoughts about being a bad veterinarian or catch yourself avoiding challenging tasks for fear that you may not be good enough at your job to achieve them. You likely do not know the true root of the imposter syndrome by just thinking it through. First, begin to notice your thoughts. Then notice the body reactions. They often feel fear. Slow this down and acknowledge that making a mistake has become the saber-tooth tiger in the room. Now notice that this is a nervous system response. The best way to address phobias is through exposure. Now, I am not telling you to go make as many mistakes as possible. I am saying notice that when you make a mistake or do not know the answer to something, it does not kill you. This allows your nervous system to calm down slowly. Reframe this as a way to learn and be better in the future, and it begins to address the fear. There will always be someone better at something than you are. In addition, you will be better at your job 10 years from now than you are now in the same way that you are better at what you do than you were 10 years ago. Allowing for some safety in the fear enables the nervous system to slow down so that the issue can be addressed.

CONCLUSION

When people complain about a symptom, my first thought process is "how was that serving you at one point?" Sometimes the symptom itself becomes the threat because people view themselves as broken because they experience symptoms. When the symptom is redefined as a neurological response to safety, which was, at one point, protective, it can allow us to view the symptoms from a different light. That simple shift can change the layers of the struggle and allow for more insight and more progress in resilience. If needed, you can use some skills to communicate to the nervous system that you are safe. As difficult as this is, it is much more effective than trying to argue with it cognitively.

This is where the age-old nature vs. nurture argument comes in. A vast majority of responses are nervous system responses that come from messages throughout our lives and as ways to protect us from things that have happened in the past. However, it is also worth acknowledging that some personality traits we are likely born with. There is a question about whether this is due to traumatized genetics or just a simple disposition. I do not know, but what I do know is that animals are born with personalities, and we are animals, so I would guess that there is some level of predisposition. We all have things we are naturally good at and things we struggle with. Some people are born with a depletion of neurotransmitters, which contributes to mental health struggles when left untreated. This has nothing to do with the life they live and everything to do with the way they are born. Some people are born with bigger emotions. We have also all lived life and had people communicate crummy things to us throughout our lives. Some more than others, but we all have some kind of nasty message sitting up there in our noggins.

As humans, we believe that if we fully understand where and why things happen, we can find an answer. This is true to some extent. The neurologists that I follow has allowed us to look at our reactions from a different perspective than we once did. We can alter our therapeutic method in a way that works with our nervous system and body so that we can make changes from the bottom up instead of trying to use our thoughts only to make changes. However, we will not be able to understand everything. Sometimes knowing where something comes from only provides us with information about its origin; it does not create any movement at all. Please notice if you get lost in this for yourself. It may be a way that your body is distracting you from the real work. See if you can be curious about your responses without understanding why you have them. It may allow more space to use the skills to the best of your ability, without the chatter of the brain.

FOOD FOR THOUGHT JOURNAL TOPIC:

Next time you notice a symptom, sticky point, or part of you that you would like to change, take some time in that moment, or maybe later on in your commute or quiet time alone, to journal.

1. Notice the symptom or reaction and describe it.

2. What is this reaction that you don't like protecting you from? What is unsafe? What is your saber-tooth tiger in this situation? *You can guess. It doesn't matter much if you get it right or wrong.*

3. Think about how it has served you as a protective mechanism, even if it doesn't make logical sense.

4. Think about ways in which it is trying to continue to protect you and no longer needs to.

5. Write a letter thanking it for the role that it has played and letting it know it can chill when it is getting in the way of things.

REFERENCES

Butler, O. *et al.* (2020). 'Trauma, treatment and Tetris: Video gaming increases hippocampal volume in male patients with combat-related posttraumatic stress disorder', *Journal of Psychiatry & Neuroscience*, 45(4), pp. 279–287. https://doi.org/10.1503/jpn.190027.

Dana, D. (2020). *Polyvagal Exercises for Safety and Connection: 50 Client-Centered Practices*. New York: W. W. Norton & Company.

Gregory, B. (2012). 'Utilizing and integrating mathematics and physics in treatment for recovery from trauma and abuse', in Gow, K. and Celinski, M. J. (eds.) *Individual Trauma: Recovering from Deep Wounds and Exploring the Potential for Renewal*. Hauppauge, NY: Nova Science Publishers, pp. 319–336.

Hagenaars, M. A., Holmes, E. A., Klaassen, F. and Elzinga, B. (2017). 'Tetris and word games lead to fewer intrusive memories when applied several days after analogue trauma', *European Journal of Psychotraumatology*, 8(sup1), 1386959. https://doi.org/10.1080/20008198.2017.1386959.

Holmes, E. A., James, E. L., Coode-Bate, T. and Deeprose, C. (2009). 'Can playing the computer game "Tetris" reduce the build-up of flashbacks for trauma? A proposal from cognitive science', *PLoS One*, 4(1), e4153.

Iyadurai, L. *et al.* (2017). 'Preventing intrusive memories after trauma via a brief intervention involving Tetris computer game play in the emergency department: a proof-of-concept randomised controlled trial', *Molecular Psychiatry*, 23(3), pp. 674–682.

Rosenberg, S. (2017). *Accessing the Healing Power of the Vagus Nerve: Self-Help Exercises for Anxiety, Depression, Trauma and Autism*. Berkeley, CA: North Atlantic Books.

CHAPTER 13
Shared Emotional States

Many of us have witnessed that a less-resilient team member can bring the rest of the team down with their reactions, negativity, and stuckness. As the burnout and poor emotion regulation spread, it can be like lobsters in a bucket pulling each other down. In the same way, a more resilient team member can create space for other people to build resilience, increasing the emotional regulation of other members of the team. You alone really can change the vibe of an entire team (assuming there are no other external barriers fighting against it). Magnetic readers have read that we have approximately three feet of a magnetic field that surrounds us and intertwines with each other (McCraty, 2004, McCarty et al. 1998, McCarty, 2017). You have felt this before when you are starting next to an anxious person, and they are making you anxious. Watching pack animals communicate and applying this to the shared emotional state, I can infer that we are likely reading micro cues from people around us about what is safe. If one person is anxious, we need to be anxious as well so that we can protect ourselves and our pack from the threat. As we subconsciously read nonverbal cues around us, we also begin to develop similar emotions to those around us. Our interactions with each other were tested by applying a cognitive test in two rooms. The participants were given a cognitive test while the administrator practiced nervous system regulation techniques, while people took the test. These participants were given a second test similar to the first, and the administrator was given cues that would activate the nervous system and create anxiety. The participants performed overwhelmingly better on the first test (Mccraty, 2004). When brain scans have been conducted around compassion, scientists have been able to see what are known as mirror neurons. Neurons are the receptors in the brain that receive and send information to the body to respond accordingly. Mirror neurons are when the neurons in one person's brain mimic those of another person's brain, even though their stimuli are different (Mikołajewska *et al.*, 2022). These mirror neurons tell us that our brains are communicating with each other and mimicking each other even when we are unaware of it.

Shared nervous systems can be particularly dangerous in a clinic where staff are burned out. The good news about this is that wellness is also contagious. If one person is regulating their nervous system in an anxious environment, the nervous systems of others in the room will also regulate. Even the slightest increase in regulation allows space for people to manage their emotions more effectively at a subconscious level.

This viewpoint is helpful for the people-pleaser or those who tend to be helpers. Managing your emotions and well-being is not just about you and how you feel. It can alter the vibe of the clinic you work in and improve the mood of those around you. If you don't do it for you, do it for your colleagues, your family members, or the patients coming in.

We refer to our ability to react to other people's emotions as attunement. While attunement may seem superficial to some, it is a very important part of how people react to each other. This can be the reaction of your team, the handler you are working with, or your partner, friend, or children. We know that people who feel seen and have conscious attunement around them perform better academically (Poulson and Fouts, 2001). You likely perform attunement very naturally with animals. When an anxious animal walks into your clinic, you are likely aware that relaxing your own body can relax the animal to an extent.

Attunement is an evolutionary structure that can be seen in all primates. It is believed that the ability to attune comes from a need to gain social acceptance and teamwork within a group of primates (Poulson and Fouts, 2001). When our emotions are extremely high, it is more difficult to regulate for attunement. When we are out of our emotional window, we become absorbed in what will keep us safe from the individual perspective and struggle with what we can do to provide teamwork. This can be especially difficult when we do not agree with the person we are working with. When someone is being a jerk, I do not always want to connect with that person on any level. However, if we regulate our own system, we are more likely to communicate effectively, validate when needed, and ultimately, we might even be heard and listened to more.

Still not buying the attunement piece? Animal-assisted therapy utilizes this attunement between animals and humans. It has been shown that touch, proximity, and interactions with animals allow for healing in traumatized individuals. Experiencing symptoms of PTSD. This is likely due to the calming effects of the dog's neurons being received by the human (Yorke, 2010). They are pack animals, we are pack animals, why wouldn't we share neurons, safety responses, and emotional space.

If attunement is contagious, how do you keep yourself from "catching grumpy" from the people around you? You can alter the vibe of the room through introspection (looking at your own body reactions and how they may be similar to the person you are interacting with) or by being more logical ("This person's brow is furrowed, they must be angry"). If you are not sure which one is easier for you, try both out and see which fits better. You can ask these questions out loud ("I notice you are angry right now") or silently in your mind. Either way, adding compassion to your interaction allows you to separate their emotions from your own so that you can see the situation from your own knowledge and values instead of from the emotions of others in the room. Using logic and curiosity allows us to pull ourselves out of the other person's emotional spiral, giving us a chance to change the vibe of the room.

One of the things that I notice within the veterinary field is that, as a field, attunement has been geared toward burnout, cynicism, and emotional disconnection. Burnout is expected and worn as a badge of honor. Grumpiness and disconnection are seen as "just the way it is." As a field, veterinary medicine tends to focus on the negative more than the positive. There is a belief that if we do not try to fix what went wrong, we will miss it and things will get worse. This feeds into the natural cynicism that comes up when we are discussing personality in the field. It is true that the negative is important; however, the positive is also important. In fact, maximizing the impact of positive events has been proven to improve well-being (Smits, 2022). If we do not create space for wellness, there will never be a change in the field.

It is also important to acknowledge that the more power and prestige you have, the more impact your emotions have on the people around you. If you are the owner of the practice, your staff will be watching you to see how they should manage their emotions. The more power you have, the more impact you have on the people around you. In the same way, if you have many people working above you who are less willing to work on their well-being, it will likely be an uphill battle for you to change the culture completely. You may be able to change some of the space you share with others, but the culture is unlikely to change without intervention from higher-ups. The importance of this contagious effect of emotions is mentioned in Ahha's white paper Stay, please

(AAHA, 2024). The number one factor that makes people want to stay is teamwork. Without knowing each other's strengths, supporting one another, and acknowledging where someone needs support, teamwork is ineffective. Supporting a team through teamwork is essential. Attunement allows us not only to regulate our own emotions but also to read the needs of others more effectively. A wonderful skill in building the team around us.

EXERCISE 13.1 Attunement

In a room of people where there may be large amounts of emotions, ask yourself, "what is mine and what is theirs" and notice what happens. You do not have to think hard or dive deep into this difficult topic.

1. Notice your felt sense in the situation. *Tight chest, lump in your throat, tight jaw, etc.*

2. Notice the other person's nonverbal cues and put words to them. "They have scrunched face" or "there muscles are tight."

3. Then go back to your own reactions, "My chest is tight."

4. Ask the felt sense (as if you are talking to something outside of yourself), "What is mine and what is theirs?"

5. Notice what happens.

FOOD FOR THOUGHT JOURNAL TOPIC:

1. How do I see attunement show up in my workplace?

2. What role do I play in the vibe of the clinic I work in?

3. Where can I apply attunement to my everyday life?

REFERENCES

American Animal Hospital Association (2024) Stay, please: Veterinary medicine has a problem—it's losing good people at an unsustainable rate. Available at: https:// www. aaha. org

McCraty, R. (2004). 'The energetic heart: Bioelectromagnetic communication within and between people', in Rosch, P. J. and Markov, M. S. (eds.) *Clinical Applications of Bioelectromagnetic Medicine.* New York: Marcel Dekker, pp. 541–562.

McCraty, R., Atkinson, M., Tomasino, D. and Tiller, W. A. (1998). 'The electricity of touch: Detection and measurement of cardiac energy exchange between people', in Pribram, K. H. (ed.) *Brain and Values: Is a Biological Science of Values Possible?* Mahcaw, NewJersey: Lawrence Erlbaum Associates, Publishers, pp. 359–379.

McCraty, R. (2017). 'New frontiers in heart rate variability and social coherence research: Techniques, technologies, and implications for improving group dynamics and outcomes', *Frontiers in Public Health*, 5, 267. https://doi.org/10.3389/fpubh. 2017.00267.

Mikołajewska, E. *et al.* (2022). 'From neuroimaging to computational modeling of burnout: The traditional versus the fuzzy approach—A review', *Applied Sciences*, 12(22), p. 11524.

Poulsen, J. and Fouts, G. (2001). 'Facilitating academic achievement through affect attunement in the classroom', *The Journal of Educational Research*, 94(3), pp. 185–190 https://doi.org/10.1080/00220670109599915.

Smits, F. (2022) *Autistic veterinary surgeons in the United Kingdom: Workplace stressors and mental wellbeing* [Master of Research Thesis, University of Nottingham]. Available at: http://eprints.nottingham.ac.uk/78517/1/14324658_Femke%20Smits_MRES%20thesis%20corrections.pdf (Accessed: 14 October 2025).

Yorke, J. (2010). 'The significance of human–animal relationships as modulators of trauma effects in children: A developmental neurobiological perspective', *Early Child Development and Care*, 180(5), pp. 559–570.

CHAPTER 14

The Skeptic

I am a big fan of a skeptic. I love it when people question what they're reading, especially when it comes to something as counterintuitive as listening to your body more than your thoughts.

It is not uncommon for people to say, "But if you can't figure it out, how do you fix it?" You actually are figuring it out by listening to your body. It just happens spontaneously and with less frantic thinking. If you have been trying to figure it out and it is not working, it might be time to try something else. If you have questions come up as I talked about the natural safety responses in the nervous system, become curious about the reactions in your own body. The only way I know how to prove this to you is for you to try. It might be uncomfortable, but give a set amount of time, maybe a few weeks to a few months, to just try to explore your body sensations, not make meaning of them, not figure them out, just to notice them. I know it's not easy. Once you have been curious about your reactions for your predetermined amount of time, you can decide if this fits your needs. If it does not, I encourage you to find some alternative coping mechanisms outside of this book. If it does, great, you learned something new about yourself. I feel confident this will work for you because I have seen it time and time again in people I work with. I do not expect you to trust it just because I say it may work.

Sometimes we feel out of control when we give up figuring it out. We have been acting in one way for so long that it has become a comfort blanket for us. Feel free to start small with the concept that feels less intimidating to you. As long as this discomfort is tolerable, that is okay, just notice that too. You may have thoughts like, "I'm doing this wrong?" or you may catch yourself planning this out in so much detail that you never actually get to the try it out part. If you are trying to notice you are doing it wrong, just notice that thought and what comes up in your body. If you notice yourself planning so much that you are not accomplishing any tasks, I encourage you just to start. Let it be imperfect. Sometimes, people even get angry at themselves or others as they try out these skills. This is actually part of the process, not interfering with the process. Notice that and then go back to your task at hand. Remember, when trying out these skills, you may notice anger and decide not to act on it; in fact, that would be pretty great practice.

I'm not going to lie. I was a skeptic of this stuff, too. I can't exactly tell you why I decided to try it out or get trained in it. I think there was a part of me that hoped I could prove it all wrong. I tried it and saw more profound changes than I had with the cognitive work I was doing before. I saw changes in myself as I started to slow down and notice. The more I dove into the world, the more it moved from "fruity woo woo stuff" to something that makes logical sense. Our spontaneous reactions have become more information for change instead of something to heal or fix.

Have you ever noticed how your body and mind react during an argument? Maybe you tell your mind that a plane ride is pretty safe, but your body is super anxious. Perhaps you know that you have a million positive Google reviews for every negative one, but you are terrified of a negative review. My logical mind says everything is day-to-day safety, but my body says, "get the hell out of here, you might die." You can start by simply noticing when an argument arises between your body and mind. Maybe it will be helpful, maybe it won't, but it is a great way to start to see if you connect with this concept.

I encourage the skeptic to stay skeptical and try some of this. I can't promise you that it's going to work for you. I can only say that it works for many people that I teach and use this with. Please let it be weird. Please let it not make sense, and try it anyway. Try it to prove me wrong, and let's just see what happens.

Take a moment and think about something you do that has delayed satisfaction. For many living in Colorado, this is considered a summit hikes or a very hard hobby. There are usually moments in these kinds of hobbies where you might say, "Why the hell do I do this?" It's not super fun along the journey. When you reach the top or complete the task, you feel great about yourself or the world. That's what we're hoping for here that delayed satisfaction. Sometimes you might get some satisfaction along the way, but the delayed satisfaction is where the real change is.

Now that I have talked you into just trying and seeing what happens, I will step aside and keep my bias out of it so as not to influence your experience. I have a whole chapter talking you into trying, so I obviously have a bias. However, from the bottom of my heart, I want you to try this out for yourself. I want you to see if it fits for you, and I want to give you permission to alter it if it does not fit for you.

FOOD FOR THOUGHT JOURNALING:

1. As you read about the nervous system where are you skeptical? Where are you curious?

2. What may get in the way of you becoming curious about how your nervous system is reacting? Develop a plan for noticing the barrier.

Building Workplace Well-Being

N ow that we understand why and how our nervous system struggles in stressful work environments, we can address building a workplace based on well-being. Once we are more grounded from a body system prospective, it is easier to move to more cognitive approaches to change. When we attempt to change before feeling grounded it can often feel frantic and be less productive. Once you have addressed your responses from a nervous system prospective you can review your values and begin develop value based work. You can also decide where acceptance is needed more than change. You can acknowledge the difficulties of expectations and decision making and begin developing a plan to make these difficult parts of the job more manageable. We can start to develop habits and skills that can build resilience to well-being in the future. While these skills often seem easier than the nervous system skills, they are often hard to carry out on a day to day basis. They take practice and messing up before they become habitual and easy to use. In many ways they are harder to apply because we are trying to apply them in a fast paced environment. Unfortunately things do not slow down so that we can use our skills. Use patients with yourself when applying the skills. Finding ways to apply them in the best way possible, while also acknowledging it is difficult to change quickly is very important with all of the concepts listed in this section. The best way to build and gain resilience to well-being struggle is to use both nervous system skills and cognitive skills in a balanced way. We need both to thrive.

Knowing Your Values and How They Can Impact Your Well-Being

Values are a simple yet complex topic that is essential to address when discussing workplace well-being. Many times when I ask people to address their top three values off the top of their heads, they are very different from the values that are exposed after exploring them.

Why would that be? Why would so many people be so very disconnected from their values that they list them differently? Often, our surface-level value system is composed of values we believe we should have. Our family system established values that they believe are the best values. The career system establishes values it thinks we should have. School established values that it feels we should have. Here we are left with values that are not authentically ours. Within the field of veterinary medicine, there is a value of being more dedicated to work above all things, care of animals coming before finances, and perfectionism with every case you treat. I then notice that when people see flaws in these values, they swing in the other direction; make sure you prioritize family life at all times, set prices high, and allow for all the mistakes that you need to. The problem is that it really does not address finding your own value system and making decisions based on what you authentically believe. Don't worry, therapists do this too; there is a reason I notice this with veterinary professionals.

Unfortunately, books are not therapy, so it would be very difficult to dive deep into your individualized personal authentic self, but we can scratch the surface of finding your authentic values, which are so essential for the following few chapters of skills and discussion.

I would like to share with you my values before you start your own. I do this because I have read many books where I close the book and try my best to apply the concepts to my life, and for some reason, I just cannot make it fit. Through reflection, I realized that all writers utilize their values to write the book. Otherwise, it would not be important enough to them to spend the time to write it. I hope that in being transparent with my values, you can see where I am coming from, ensure that my values do not impact your values, and use my own journey to find my values throughout the chapter of this book. Here are some of my strongest values:

Authenticity: This is a value that I learned to cherish later in life and which is one of my very core values. I come from a family culture where fallibility should never be shown. Any personal or family flaws are promptly pushed under a huge rug, never to be discussed again. Through my own personal work, I learned that authenticity allows for a deeper connection, more powerful decision-making, and expanding growth for me personally.

Accessibility: Boy, has this one been challenged throughout my life as a business owner. Coaches everywhere tell me I should drop all insurance, raise my prices, and make a set schedule. Through a ton of soul searching, I realized that when I run from a perspective of accessibility, which is extremely important to me, creative solutions, expanded offerings, and a deeper listening to those receiving my services become apparent. There are still times my price does not fit a person's needs or someone is unable to work with my schedule, but when I am coming from big picture equity (which includes my needs as well), I notice myself thriving.

Introspection: That's what this whole book is about. Looking within ourselves in the deepest of ways to find personal growth, healing, and (here is that word again) authenticity. While looking at the outside world for changes is essential as well, my work is geared more toward introspection.

Flexibility: As a writer, I often notice myself using "yes, buts" or permission for people to connect without doing exactly what I am saying. This is because a strong value of mine is flexibility. I love to provide space for people to find what works for them. Use their creativity to modify stuff to meet their own goals and objectives. If one thing doesn't work, oh well, move on to another.

As you start to explore your own values, I recommend you take some time here. The more connected you are to your values, the more likely you are to trust your own decisions and reactions (Brown, 2015. You may have to return to this section to check back in on them a few times before you feel thoroughly grounded in them.

EXERCISE 15.1 Defining your values

---

1. Quickly scan *Figure 15.1*—notice which ones make you smile and which ones make you frown.

2. Go through the list again. Notice which values you are NOT allowed to have. Money may be the root of all evil in your family's belief, or power comes with meanness.

3. Go through the list again, point out the values you are supposed to have. Blood is thicker than water, or work hard/play hard.
   A. *These three steps allow you to become more familiar with the list and create space to find your values through the messages and shoulds that you may hold.*

2. Go through the list in *Figure 15.1* again. Identify your top 5–10 values from the list. This could be some from the list of ones you are not supposed to have or none from the ones you are supposed to have.

As you go through the list this time, ask yourself:

   A. What is important for me to teach my children *we generally want our children to be good people, which we will define from our value system?*
   B. What gets me agitated? *This can help you identify what your values are not. When* *people agitate us, they are usually acting outside of our value system.*
   C. If you had a magic wand, what would you want your world to look like? Which values fit that world?
   D. What characteristics do people you look up to have?

5. Check in with your body system as you label your five values. Where do you feel calmest when you picture yourself living life from each value? *Note: just because you have a feeling of calm does not mean it is a good value, and just because you have some disgust does not mean it is a bad value. However, checking in with what you do feel allows you to explore what fits better. When you slow down and notice your reactions, it becomes easier to identify why you feel the way you do. For instance, if you are feeling nervous about living by a value because it is new to you, when you notice the nervousness in your body system, you start to notice that the feeling is not because the value is wrong; it is simply because the value is new.*

6. Journal about each value you chose and what it means to you and your lifestyle. It is okay if the process of free-flow journaling actually changes your top values.

Achievement	Honesty	Compassion	Dedication	Hard-working
Adventure	Physical beauty	Competition	Career	Physical health
Authenticity	Visibility	Intellect	Legacy	Spirituality
Change	Stability	Predictability	Influence	Play
Cynicism	Safety	Stoicism	Glamor	Order
Courage	Uniqueness	Quality	Fairness	Freedom
Excellence	Relaxation	Self-care	Comfort	Connection
Extrospection	Independence	Integrity	Planning ahead	Perfection
Financial success	Core family	Community	Friendship	Mental well-being
Flexibility	Giving	Structure	Equity	Self-worth
Justice	Extended family	Fame	Contribution	Consideration
Leadership	Being humble	Taking responsibility	Being a change agent	Challenge
Perseverance	Relaxation	Tenacity	Bravery	Energy
Power	Acceptance of others	Responsibility	Introspection	Present day
Ritual	Flexibility	Conformity	Curiosity	Structure
Simplicity	Efficiency	Accessibility	Self-awareness	Willingness

FIGURE 15.1   A list of values to be used to assist in identifying values.

REFERENCE

Brown, B. (2015). *Daring Greatly: How the Courage to be Vulnerable Transforms the Way We Live, Love, Parent, and Lead.* New York: Avery, an Imprint of Penguin Random House.

CHAPTER 16

When Life Gives You Lemons....Just Notice them (Acceptance)

Acceptance has been such a widely used word in the world of well-being, but I would like to define it through the lens of deep acceptance. Deep acceptance can be found in many therapies, including Dr. Marsha Linehan's Dialectical Behavioral Therapy and Dr. Steven Hayes' Acceptance and Commitment Therapy. I want to preface this by saying that, within this definition, acceptance is often not a comfortable experience. The goal is not to be happy about what is happening. Sometimes acceptance is used as a way to think about the positive or force yourself to be joyful. This often does not work because there are things in life that are just plain uncomfortable. When you allow space for the painful realities with deep acceptance, you can find effective solutions. Imagine yourself pushing up against a wall. How hard do you have to press for it to move? There are many times in our lives when we push up against something that will not move. We have thoughts about fairness, the way things should be, or what we don't like about our job or our life. In these moments, our body feels like a toddler throwing a temper tantrum. Maybe we don't like that cynicism is praised in the field of veterinary medicine, or that our boss does not value family life in the same way we do, or that politics are leaned against our own belief and value system. It can really make us miserable to focus on the parts of life that we dislike. When we are pushing up against the wall of change, it can lead to a spiral of thoughts, feelings of being stuck, and unresolvable anger. It creates misery.

Signs that you are trying to change something that cannot be changed (pushing up against the wall):

- Ruminating thoughts about something being unfair

- Feeling "stuck in the mud" about a concept

- Thoughts such as "It shouldn't be this way," or "It's not fair"

- Misery about a specific situation or concept

When we work toward deep acceptance, we do not work toward comfort or agreement with a situation. We work toward recognition of the facts. We acknowledge that the facts are sometimes painful. We recognize that not all discomfort can be changed.

I often get the argument, "But we have to fight for what is wrong to create change." I wholeheartedly agree with this. Please do not stop fighting (If this is within your value system). However, many times we cannot see the avenue toward change until we have a deep acceptance of the facts.

For example, *you continue to argue and disagree with your boss about how family should be valued in the workplace. She continues to hold the ground that work should come first. Every time she enacts a new policy that gets in the way of your family life, you begin fuming. You complain to your partner, your colleagues, and anyone who will hear you. You cannot stop thinking about how toxic the workplace is. You have given her the research studies, talked with her about the importance of work–life balance, and gotten downright mad at her, but nothing is shifting. You work toward acceptance. You follow some of the steps listed below. It is really very sad to you that she runs her practice this way and that so many people suffer. You feel disheartened by the field, as this is a common trend in larger companies. You allow yourself the sadness and grief that comes with what you wish was not true. As you continue in this process, you begin to research jobs in your community. You decide to apply for a position at a smaller clinic that has a flexible vacation policy. You interview and really like the vibe. You feel nervous, fearing that it will be more of the same, but you give it a shot.*

The problem-solving that comes after acceptance is not always to leave a position or the field. Sometimes, it is a path toward education and reform. Whatever you decide to do, it will likely feel more grounded than it would if it were coming from a place of rejection of reality. Within acceptance, as painful as something is, we can turn down our emotions just enough to find a path toward productive problem-solving. It creates space to find a way to live in reality. Sometimes that means an avenue toward change. Sometimes it allows us to remember a coping mechanism. I am reiterating once again that our systems are smart; we just need to give them space to work. This often means finding a way to push all our junk aside for a moment, or better yet, work through it. This concept allows this to happen.

Acceptance is way easier said than done. We do not want the painful thing to be true. Who would? We may find acceptance in one moment, and the next go back to wanting to stomp our feet and throw things. Just because acceptance comes in and out does not mean you are doing this wrong. You will likely have to go back to acceptance a million times. This is because acceptance is hard, not because you are doing it wrong.

Think about this as if it were a scale, as is portrayed in Figure 16.1. If we lean too much toward acceptance, the scale will not be even, and we may end up sitting on our hands. If we lean too much toward change, the scale will not be even, and we will feel stuck, unable to see what can change and what stands firm. The ideal place is to have equal amounts of change and acceptance.

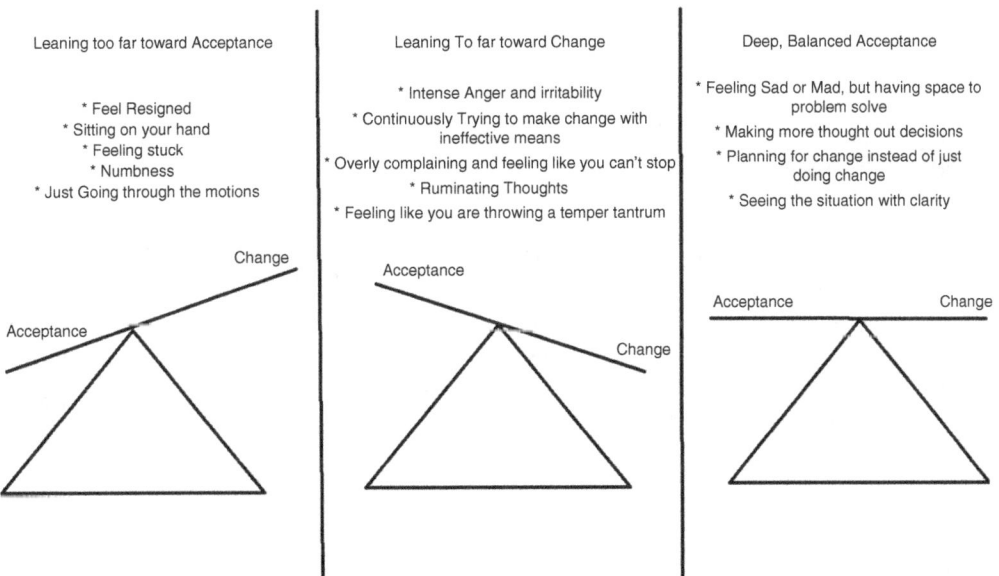

FIGURE 16.1 Shows how you may feel when you are focused more on acceptance or change and how you may feel when there is a greater balance.

Through true acceptance, we find an ability to find movement around a situation through spontaneous problem-solving vs. trying to power through it or wallowing in misery. It allows us to decide what is worth the fight and how to fight well instead of stomping our feet and yelling (on the inside, and on the outside).

Whether you are religious or not, the idea of acceptance often reminds people of the Serenity Prayer:

Grant me the Serenity to accept the things I cannot change, courage to change the things I can, and Wisdom to know the difference. **Reinhold Neibuhr**

Some may read this as a prayer, some may read this as a quote, some may reject it all altogether, but it really consolidated the concept of acceptance.

EXERCISES THAT HELP US MOVE TOWARD ACCEPTANCE

EXERCISE 16.1 | Willing hands/accepting hands

One step toward acceptance is to think of a situation with willing hands. I have seen and heard concepts about the way that we sit across several different important avenues. In yoga classes, I hear instructors refer to open hands as openness and closed hands as being grounded. Therapy techniques like Dialectical Behavioral Therapy discuss it as a technique toward acceptance. I personally used to use it when I worked in an agency, when staff meetings felt frivolous or outside of my value system. It seems way too simple to work sometimes, but I encourage you to try it out and see if it works for you.

1. Sit with your palms faced up.

2. Think about or hold an image of the thing that you are stuck in or upset about.

3. Notice what happens. Maybe you feel different, maybe the image doesn't seem so big, and maybe you become sad. Just notice.

4. If you get stuck in ruminating thoughts, stop and do something else. If you notice it is painful, allow for the emotion as much as you are able to tolerate. You may have to start with moments of this practice at a time if the emotion is so painful that it is difficult to tolerate.

5. Move on with life after doing this for a few moments at a time.

Source: Linehan, 2015.

EXERCISE 16.2 | Neutral face

Your face holds so many of your emotions. It is the way we communicate with each other non-verbally. When someone has a furrowed brow, you know that they are mad. When someone frowns, you know they are sad, and when someone smiles, you know they are happy. Our facial expressions are often spontaneous. Sometimes, we do not even know we are making them. Sometimes we can work backward and change our expression to work toward our next steps.

1. Let your face relax into a neutral position. I like to rub my hands down my face, dragging it down to relax it.

2. Bring your fingers to the corner of your lips and push them to a straight line. Not frowning, no smiling, just straight. Think Mona Lisa.

3. Release your fingers and think about the thing you are stuck in or upset about in this neutral position.

4. Notice if your attitude or thoughts change. They may or may not just allow it to be.

Source: Linehan, 2015.

EXERCISE 16.3   Thought distancing

When we are rejecting reality, our thoughts hold so much weight that it can be difficult to move toward anything. Sometimes they ruminate so much that it is difficult to find any space toward acceptance. When we turn down our thoughts in this way, it is often more likely that we can move toward acceptance.

1. Acknowledge the thing that you are stuck on and put words to it.

2. Find some silly way to help the thought have less meaning. Here are some ideas:
   a. Sing the concept in the tune of a children's song
   b. Say the idea in several different silly voices

c. Repeat a word or a few words about the idea several times in your head until it loses its meaning
d. Give the concept a name and acknowledge that's just .... When the thoughts come in. (Example: *The world is going to end.... Oh, that's just my anxiety.*)

3. Check in on the concept. See if it still has the same misery associated with it. Notice if anything has changed or if it is the same.

EXERCISE 16.4   Acceptance through mindfulness of emotions

In the last chapter, I spoke often about the body knowing more than the mind due to nervous system responses. This exercise speaks to this concept in the context of acceptance. Some people may struggle with this. If you try it and just can't find where it is in your body, move on to the journaling or a different skill.

1. Think about the concept that you know is difficult to accept, and sit with it for a moment. Some people visualize an interaction that symbolizes it, some just think about the concept itself. Whatever elicits the uncomfortable emotions for you, do it.

2. Notice what you feel in your body.
   a. What is your facial expression? Where is your face tight or scrunched?
   b. How are you sitting when you think about it? Hunched over? Tight? Crossed arms?

c. What do you notice inside your body? Where are you tight, jittery, warm, or feel any other sensation?

3. Bring your attention to this sensation. Can you notice any details in it that you have not noticed before?

4. Breathe into this sensation. You may notice thoughts come in; just let them and go back to the sensation itself.

5. Notice if there are shifts or changes in the sensation, thoughts, or intensity as you give this sensation awareness.

6. Go back to the distress. Has it changed or is it the same?

EXERCISE 16.5	Effective list making

Sometimes, making small changes in our lives can allow space for us to accept in a more logical way. Movement feels good and can empower us to notice other places we can move. This skill/journal prompt is designed to help you move in the small ways you are capable of moving so that you can naturally move toward acceptance.

1. Make a list of all the things that frustrate you or worry you. Make the list as big as you possibly can. If it is absurd, add it; if it is very valid, add it. In this step, you are not analyzing or figuring anything out; you are only listing.

2. Go through and cross out the items that are objectively silly worries. It is not uncommon to have these.

3. Go through the list and circle the items that are valid (i.e., things I should worry about, it has the potential to be a threat to safety or values).

4. Go back through the circled items and highlight the items that you have power over and can change.

5. Pick one or two of the highlighted items.

6. List three **realistic** tasks you can do today to work toward a resolution. It may be tempting to be an overachiever here, but pull back those reins. You can go back and make more tasks later if you need to. You can make bigger and broader goals another day. These are small, realistic tasks.

7. Set a timer for a time to check in. See if you followed through with those tasks. If you did great, do it again next time you feel flustered (or tomorrow if that's all the time right now). If you did not follow through, move to the next step.

8. Re-read the tasks. Are you capable of following through with them? If they were too big, make them smaller. If they were not realistic, rewrite them. No excuses allowed here. If you didn't have time, that means it is too big. The key here is to be as realistic as possible, given your current life and schedule. If you brainstorm ways to make it more realistic and notice that you have a strong avoidance, no matter how large it is. Notice that and find the level of it that is challenging, but the avoidance is tolerable. *Example: I made the goal to find something I did well in the day while I drive home from work. I forgot for two days in a row. When I reviewed it, it was difficult to make it more achievable. I have the time, I am driving anyway. I didn't forget; I set an alarm. I simply do not want to do it. I decided to reframe this skill for now and explored what I learned today. I still did not want to do it. I want to zone out and listen to my tunes. I feel capable of reflecting on what I've learned. I can follow through with this and I notice that I worry less about my skills at work. I followed through and noticed that my view of the day changed. Eventually, I add the task of noticing what I did well today. It feels more achievable after I've had a chance to apply what I've learned for a few days.*

9. Try again and see what the new tasks look like. Repeat steps 5 and 6 as many times as you can. If you start getting defeated, ask someone else to review it and help you find some realistic steps. Failure to complete the tasks is not designed to make you feel worse about yourself or defeated. It is designed to give you more information about what needs to be accepted and what parts of your life you can change.

Warning about acceptance: We do not always like the answer. Oftentimes, the concept we are accepting is painful, which is why we have a desire not to accept it. Sometimes the change portion is also uncomfortable. This is why we have chosen not to move toward the change. Allow some space for the discomfort and decide if it is worth it. This process can allow you to slow this down in order to make a move that is likely to be the best move for you.

REFERENCES

Hayes, S. C., Strosahl, K. D. and Wilson, K. G. (2012). *Acceptance and Commitment Therapy: The Process and Practice of Mindful Change* (2nd ed.). New York: American Psychological Association.

Linehan, M. M. (2015). *DBT® Skills Training Handouts and Worksheets* (2nd ed.). New York: The Guilford Press.

CHAPTER 17

Connection

When mental well-being and mental health peak their heads out of the sand, sometimes shame sneaks in with them. Some of this comes with the stigma of mental well-being, and some comes from old messages about what we should feel, act, and do in our lives. Whatever the origin of the shame, when it settles in, we often have the urge to isolate. Conscious or unconscious shame communicates that we are a bad person, and we want to protect others from our "badness." It is difficult to tell people about our struggles, and we worry we will either infect them with our struggles, be a burden, or send some other message that keeps us hiding the secret that many people are hiding beside us. Many times, the urge to disconnect is spontaneous, and we don't even think about the fact that it is happening. The problem is that connection is not only important, but it is essential. We are pack animals; we need to connect and communicate with each other to thrive as a community.

Many times, when someone is struggling, they naturally begin to disconnect. This can look like keeping their struggle internal and talking to no one, pushing people away by ignoring them, or becoming irritable toward them, or all around trying to pick yourself up by your bootstraps all by yourself. Disconnection can also take the form of compassion fatigue (feeling cold toward situations that would usually foster deep emotions). Disconnect is a natural coping mechanism we develop, designed to protect us. Our subconscious fears that someone may find out this struggle that "we shouldn't have" and may judge us for it. While disconnecting may seem glorious to those who are feeling large emotions or fed up with people, it has a lot of destructive properties. When our body develops a protective coping mechanism, it has a difficult time deciding when to use it and when not to. You may decide to disconnect from handlers only. You have held too many of their emotions over time and hope that disconnection will solve the problem. Over time, disconnection begins to bleed into day-to-day life. When the system hopes to disconnect from only handlers, it starts to disconnect from colleagues, and eventually it bleeds over to friends, family, and loved ones. This leads to an isolating lifestyle where work becomes the main purpose. When work becomes challenging and this is one's sole purpose, it can really do a number on well-being.

If you are reading this and thinking, "Well, I am an introvert, so I do not need connection." I would like to challenge you. An introvert gains energy from being alone and often problem-solves internally before asking for help, but an introvert still needs connection. Sometimes this connection is simply someone sitting beside them in silence, but it is still a connection. When one is struggling to connect, they may mislabel themselves as an introvert. Some people are introverted and also avoid some emotions or thoughts through isolation. Others isolate as a protective mechanism and define themselves as introverts because being by themselves is more comfortable. When we dig deeper, we find that they are actually avoiding judgment, social anxiety, or something else uncomfortable, and actually gain energy from being around others. Even if you gain energy by being by yourself, you also need people around you in some way, shape, form, or fashion. This looks different for everyone. I challenge you to explore what this means for you.

When I refer to a need for connection, people sometimes assume I mean being deeply vulnerable with another person. While this could be true, it could also be as simple as standing beside someone, smiling at someone, or otherwise feeling a sense of shared community. Connection does not have to be around sharing the things that make you feel ashamed or your deepest, darkest secrets. While this can be helpful with trusted people, it is not the only way to connect. Sometimes connection involves sitting beside someone while you work, letting someone know you care, and them doing the same, giving a small gift to someone (not necessarily monetary), or any other items I list below. If a connection is wanted but difficult, start small and notice what happens when you attempt to connect, then add more connections as you become more comfortable.

It would be remiss of me to mention the need for connection without also acknowledging how stinking hard it is to gain deep connection with new people in adult life. Throughout school (including higher education), we are around people and often have some commonality that we can talk about. In adult life, we are usually spread out, and finding something in common takes uncomfortable small talk. If you are someone reading this section who is feeling lonely because you do not have friends, start with the various forms of connection that are less about making friends. If you make friends along the way, great, but the intention of this exercise right now is simply to practice connection even when it is not the connection you necessarily crave.

While friendship is comforting and sometimes needed, the connection we are talking about in this moment is more of an opening of the eyes to notice that we are not alone on this planet. Friendship making comes later, when you are more comfortable.

VARIOUS LEVELS OF CONNECTION

When we begin to disconnect, we do not just disconnect from people, although this is the disconnection that can be the most obvious. We also start to disconnect from ourselves. This would manifest as feeling numb to emotions, being unable to label internal reactions to emotions and events, being unsure of our values, feeling like you are going through the motions of life, or being unable to find joy in activities you once found enjoyable. This happens when the body interprets all responses from the body as unsafe. When we disconnect from ourselves and others, we also disconnect from the world around us. You may overlook details as you once did. Disconnection from nature and the world is harder to notice than the other two.

When you disconnect from people, you may disconnect in multiple layers. Disconnection can happen to the outer community as a whole. You may not know how you fit in with the world around you. You may feel like you are on an island when you interact with people in public. You may disconnect from other people closer to you. You may feel like you just cannot feel a connection with loved ones, family, partners, or kids.

You may feel connected to one or all of these layers. Many times, the layers start to blend, creating a deeper disconnection the longer you go. If you are feeling very disconnected from any part of your world, it is recommended to exercise patience with the skills discussed. Your nervous system has labeled connections as dangerous for one reason or another. It believes that if you are connected, you may become hurt or hurt others. It may also worry you that you may feel emotions

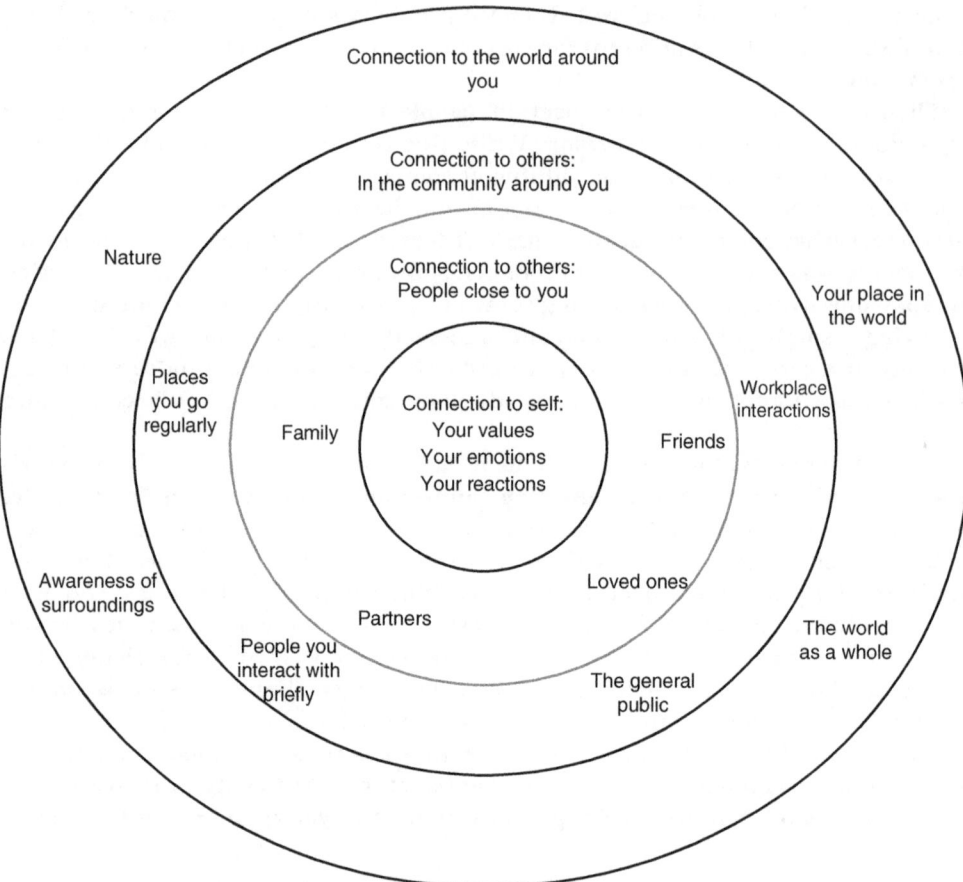

FIGURE 17.1 Various levels of connection starting with connection to self, including values, emotions, and reactions. Connection to people close to you, like family, friends, loved ones, and partners. Connection to your community, which is all the people you interact with, and connection with the world.

you would prefer to avoid. Start small with the strategies discussed and allow yourself to notice small changes that can work toward a bigger shift toward connection.

By working toward connection at various levels, we can start to build safety within our bodily system, ultimately leading to a deeper connection with ourselves and others. By defining the levels of connection, we can find the safest way to connect, without feeling overwhelmed by the world around us. The various levels can also feel less intimate to someone who is feeling disconnected. It may feel like connecting to nature is not related, but the more you connect to the small things, the easier it is to begin connecting to the bigger things (usually other humans). In Figure 17.1, you can see the various levels of connection and how they relate to your core self. As you notice disconnection in each layer and work toward a greater connection, they all work together.

EXERCISE 17.1   Finding connection through nature

Connection to Nature

The first level to connect to is nature. This level is often overlooked when discussing connection. However, for many, it is the safest way to connect. Nature tends to be safer than people or ourselves. It generally cannot hurt us (yes, I know there are many places nature can hurt us on a grander scale, a leaf you are noticing will not hurt you). The connection with nature allows a small avenue of safety that can lead to a grander connection in the future. The process of connection with nature can be awkward and clunky at first, especially if you are not used to noticing nature, or you are extremely disconnected. That is okay. Let it be awkward and clunky.

You can also join an online community doing the challenge with you, which may create even more connections.

- Find a detail you have not noticed before. As you notice this detail, start to notice something smaller, continuing to find the detail that is as small as you can. This can be a leaf, a dew drop, a bug, the bark of a tree, anything that interests you. *Example: There is a leaf lying in an interesting way on the ground. Its coloring is interesting. I notice that the veins in the leaf make a neat pattern. I notice that there is a dew drop on the leaf. I notice the dew drop shows a reflection.*

- Go on a walk and challenge yourself to notice a detail in nature you have not noticed before or have not noticed in a long time. *Example: That tree is bent funny, there are flowers over there I never noticed, the bark of that tree makes a neat pattern, etc.*

- Pick a color. Go on a walk and see how many shades of that color you can find in plants.

- Find something that is tactically interesting to you. A flower, a leaf, a stick, or bark are all examples. Notice what it feels like in your hand. Give words to the texture. Notice what it feels like if you rip it, scrunch it, etc.

- Lie on the ground and notice what feels like under you. Notice the ground holding you up, cooling or warming you, and being a structure for your day-to-day life. Notice where your body touches the ground, and the ground is holding you up.

- As you are lying on the ground, notice the clouds as they float above you. Become aware of the various details in the cloud.

- Notice what it feels like for your foot to touch the ground when you are walking. Notice the earth holding you up and notice your feet responding to this.

- Climb to a high spot (mountain, hill, or structure). Look around at the landscape.

- Sit by a river. Notice what you smell, then move to hear, feel, and see. Take your time noticing what it feels like to sit beside flowing water.

- Grow a plant from a seed. Be aware of all the stages the plant goes through and the details of each stage. Nurture the plant.

- Sit by a tree. Notice the details of the trunk. Move out and notice the details of the branches, then notice the details of the leaves, eventually being aware of the whole tree.

EXERCISE 17.2	Finding Connection to Self

For some people, connection to self is the next step and safer than connection to other people. Others find connection to other people safer than connection to themselves. Some people prefer to start with this and move to nature next. Whether you are doing this step first, second, or third, here are some ways you can begin to connect with yourself.

- Notice your fingerprints. Where are they soft, where are the rough? Notice how the nail feels different from the pad of the finger. Notice if you can feel the pattern in your fingerprint.

- Rub your hands together. Notice what happens as you begin to create heat with the friction of your hands. Try this fast, then try this slow, and notice the difference. Notice how your hands feel. Start to rub her arms and face as if you are removing something yucky from them. Do you feel the same, do you wake up a little, or do you feel more tired?

- Notice how you naturally sit. What parts of your body touch the chair, and where is the space? What parts of your body touch each other, and where is there space? Where is there pressure on the seat or floor? What does it feel like for your body to feel this pressure? Alter the way you are sitting and notice what is different.

- Ask yourself what you notice inside your body. I like to picture a black light going over my body and highlighting tension, tightness, and unusual sensations. You do not have to focus on the reasons for an uncomfortable sensation; it can just be a sensation. Send your focus to a sensation in the body and notice the details of this sensation.

- Notice your natural breath. Where does it start? Where does it stop? Are there any catches? Does your inhale feel different than your exhale? Expand your breath just a little deeper. How does this feel different?

EXERCISE 17.3	Connection to others

- Go to the grocery store at the same time each week and see if you feel familiar faces.

- Join a class or a hobby you are interested in (for the knowledge, but you also get community). It is especially helpful if it is a place you can show up each week with the same people. You do not have to make friends in class; it is simply about being a part of something while learning a skill.

- Give a small gift to some strangers each day. Check out Exercise 17.3.

- Notice the neighbors you see often and how you interact with them. This does not have to be huge, just a notice.

- When you are in CE events (virtual or in person), notice the number of people in the room interested in the same things that you are.

- As you calm your nervous system, take a moment to notice the people around you. Notice if they respond or act differently. Notice if they are calmer as well. No one has to know you are doing this.

- Give a 30-second hug to a loved one. Let it be weird. Giggle if you have to.

- Try out vulnerability. Maybe start small with something less scary. Make sure to try this out with someone more likely to be supportive and less likely to be critical.

- Notice people around you when running errands, and recognize that there is a world going on around you.

- Ask a friend, loved one, or colleague how they are doing and practice very active listening. Notice what happens in your body as they tell the story.

EXERCISE 17.4   29 days of giving

I am taking this exercise directly from the book *29 Gifts: How a Month of Giving Can Change Your Life* by Cami Walker and the movement of 29 Gifts (Walker 2010). I have done this challenge even though I am a natural giver. In fact, sometimes I give a little too much. This speaks to my strong value of community. I did not expect to get as much out of it, since I already gave, but I was very wrong. I gained a deeper connection to the world that is going on around me. I started to notice how people give to me, allowing space for mutual connection. Even basic places like the grocery store felt more connected than they had before. Creating the intention to complete the challenge creates a natural connection to both self and others.

The challenge is that you will give something to someone for 29 days. This does not have to be financial in any way. It could be a gift, a service, or a smile. All things count. The key to this challenge is that if you miss a day, start over at one. The second key piece is that you track the 29 days. You journal about what you did and how you are feeling. Full disclosure, my journal was a list on my phone that gave a basic description of what I did and a few words about how I felt. One day, I will do the challenge with more in-depth journaling. If you choose to do this challenge, I encourage you to make it achievable for you. However, including the key components is still important. The main pieces are: You do the challenge for 29 days, if you miss a day, you start over, and journal or track in some way.

Gifts can be:

- Give someone a compliment
- Open the door for someone
- Let someone in when traffic is bad
- Smile at someone
- Donate to a cause you care about
- Pay for the next person in line at your favorite coffee shop
- Put a funny note on someone's car or desk
- Use the in person checkout line and ask how the person's day is while you listen
- Tell someone they did a good job when you believe they did

- Let someone in in traffic
- Give some food to a food pantry
- Reach out to someone who may need it
- Volunteer for something you feel strongly about
- Ask to help someone who has a heavy load they are carrying
- Give your time to someone, even if you are busy
- Leave some cash somewhere people can find it (in the vending machine, etc.)
- Ask someone if you can cover for them while they take a break
- Make a cup of tea or coffee for someone
- Leave a positive review for a small business
- Make some treats and share them with your clinic or community group around you
- Return your shopping cart to the store instead of leaving it in the parking lot
- Let someone who looks like they are in a hurry cut you in line
- Make a meal for someone who might need it
- Plant pollinator-friendly flowers
- Send someone a handwritten letter
- Put a dollar or two in someone's coat pocket (who doesn't like finding free money in their pocket?)
- Tell a manager that an employee is doing a good job
- Send a gratitude email to a colleague who you see working very hard
- Pick up some trash on your walk
- Mow someone's lawn or shovel someone's driveway
- Clean out your books and donate them to the library
- Send inspirational quotes or stories to a friend
- Think about something that made you feel good that someone else did, and do it for someone else

When the conversation is over, it can be tempting to ruminate about the audacity of the other person and the way that they treated you. This is the body's way of validating itself. However, it can create complexity in future conversations throughout the day. You may become so agitated by this one person that you become irritable with other undeserving individuals. Your body system may perceive everything that is said to you as aggressive because it is on guard, waiting to fight others who cross your boundaries. If you find yourself so agitated that it is difficult to go on with your day in the best way possible, I recommend this exercise.

REFERENCE

Walker, C. (2010). *29 Gifts: How a Month of Giving can Change Your Life*. Boston, MA: Da Capo Life-long Books.

Communication

The need for basic communication in the field of veterinary medicine is not ignored. It is all over the place at conferences and trainings. In fact, issues with communication with handlers are often referred to as the most significant stressor for those in the veterinary field (Stetina and Krouzecky, 2022), and most people I speak with would agree. You may have learned the correct way to have conversations with handlers, and hopefully have learned how to talk to each other as well. The problem becomes when these concepts are easier said than done. Many times, communication struggles happened within heightened emotions, activating the nervous system. When someone is yelling or attacking our career, we feel threatened and want to defend ourselves. Sometimes it feels like you are the only one who is responsible for managing her emotions, and everyone else can mistreat you. It doesn't feel fair. In this chapter, we will learn how to manage our emotions so that others can manage theirs as well. A veterinary clinic is full of emotions from animals, handlers, and staff. Even one person being grounded can help to ground everyone around. Even though it is not fair that emotions are left up to you, do it anyway and see what happens. I wish I could make a requirement that people must learn to regulate emotions before walking into a clinic, but unfortunately, the world is not there yet.

People are going to trigger your safety response. They just are. They will hit that nerve that makes you feel unsafe. It may be questioning your knowledge or payment structure, or both. Everyone has things that set them off and make them want to fight the bear. The problem is, left untreated, you will bounce so far out of your window of feelings that you will be worried about defending yourself. Your brain will have to choose between the logical part of the brain and the part of the brain that is responding to safety. Because you will feel unsafe in the interactions, it will be harder to use the problem-solving, logical part of your brain. You must be grounded to be good at communication. I know this is annoying. It can feel invalidating to have to work hard to ground and respond appropriately when the other person does not have to. I wish I could make them do the same, but they are not the ones reading this book. Please know that, as hard as this is, it is much easier to leave a conversation knowing you handled it well than to leave a conversation wishing you had said something you didn't.

I have heard veterinarians report that it feels like an abusive relationship, where they are required to take verbal abuse without defending themselves. I actually hope you do not just take verbal abuse. No one deserves to be treated with verbal abuse. I give you full permission to leave the room if someone is excessively angry, and let them know you will be back in 5 minutes. As long as your clinic allows it, I also recommend that you inform verbally aggressive handlers of alternative places they can take their pet for services, as you will not tolerate this behavior. Providing referrals while asking a client to leave strikes a balance between maintaining customer service and respecting boundaries. I recommend using the following techniques before reaching this point.

This is a worst-case scenario. It is for the jerkiest of jerks. It is worth the bad review, the lost customer, or whatever fear you have that keeps you from asking this person to leave. If you use all the skills you have and nothing is working, you are being mistreated, and you do not deserve to be mistreated.

EXERCISE 18.1	Recognize your own blue flags

As you monitor your nervous system with the skills discussed in this book, you may notice that specific body reactions communicate things consistently. An example may be that you start to notice a tightened shoulder or neck muscle that is not just a result of bad posture, but also comes up every time you feel like others are judging you. You may notice your chest feels tight every time you are working with an aggressive dog. These routine body system responses can become quick information for you when in difficult conversations. I call them blue flags because they are designed to give information. These are not bad, they are great information for knowing what you need.

As you begin to notice these blue flags, you can be more prepared when walking into an exam room. A few micro-moments a day, follow these steps:

1. Pick a situation that might be difficult for you and think about it.

2. Ask: What thoughts are spontaneously coming to mind? *We are not assessing whether the thoughts are valid, helpful, or otherwise in this moment, just that they are present.* If your mind moves so fast, you are unsure of what you are thinking, try to catch just one thought that's mixed into the chaos.

3. Check in on your physiological responses. If you are a visual person, you can picture a black light scanning your entire body, highlighting tensions, tight spots, or unusual sensations. If you are not visual, just pick some sections and see how they feel. (Is there anything in my stomach? What about my chest? Do my shoulders feel anything? Etc.) Right now, we are not doing anything with them, just noticing them

4. Use this thought or body sensation as a time to check-in, next time it comes up.

5. Next time the thought and/or body sensation comes up, ask "what is going on around me." Is there a type of handler I am about to see or just saw? Is there a specific temperament or breed of animal I just saw? Did someone ask me for something annoying?

6. Exhale and go back to work. We are just building curiosity and noticing patterns.

7. As you start to notice patterns, you can begin labeling the sensation, which naturally turns down the response. *Example: each time a handler comes in who is a tall male, you notice your body tenses before entering the exam room. Now that you labeled this response, you notice the person in the exam room and your body getting tight, and you say, "Oh yeah, that is **just** my anxiety responding." The just is important here because it separates it from being very true or a big emotion. It is **just** what it is.*

Doing this regularly, you will start to notice some of these blue flags for you. This information allows you to ground yourself in whatever way you need for specific appointments that have the potential to throw you into a place where it is difficult to communicate your needs. A simple awareness that a thought or body sensation has come up allows you to ground more effectively and thus become more effective in your communication despite the stress.

VALIDATION

Validation is the act of seeking out where the other person might be coming from, even if you disagree with their perspective. "I see you feel/believe/think.... And this is what is important for me to add," Feels better to everyone than, "nope, you need to listen to me."

Many people misinterpret validation as belittling oneself for the sake of the argument or allowing the person to get their way simply to defuse the situation. I am not encouraging you to agree with them; I am merely encouraging you to consider their point of view. The benefits of this skill are twofold. It grounds you, as it requires logical thought and allows for more effective communication, because people want to be heard, even if you disagree with them. Reflecting on what you think they may be feeling can often defuse the situation. *Example: I can see you are angry, and I get it. When money is involved, it is usually stressful. However, this is our price for services.*

I want to be clear, it does not always work. Sometimes someone is so mad they snap back with "yes, of course I am angry you are terrible" or some variation of that. We are trying our best to communicate with the person who is capable of calming their nervous system enough to have communication. We have no control over the person who is not capable of this. Ultimately, we cannot control the person on the receiving end of the conversation. Even if the other person is not capable, these skills can allow you to leave the conversation knowing that you did everything you could to defuse the situation appropriately.

EXERCISE 18.2 Validation

Sometimes in the moment, it is difficult to work through the steps of validation. I encourage you to try it at whatever level you are capable of. Even if you go through these steps after the conversation is over, you may not be able to use the skill in that conversation, but you are more likely to use it in future conversations that you have.

Ask yourself:

1. What is this person scared of?

2. What might he, she, or they be activated by that they are not saying? If I were in their shoes and believed what they believed, what would I be thinking and feeling?

3. What emotion might they be feeling in this moment?

4. What do I notice in their body language? (Tight brow, shoulders moved up, pulled forward, etc.).

5. What do they need me to hear?

6. Say the validation: "I can see you are frustrated with this news".... If you get it wrong, that's okay; you can validate this as well. *For example:*
   "I can see that you are frustrated right now."
   "I am not frustrated, I am angry."
   "Yes, it makes me angry when people I feel like don't hear me as well. I want you to know that I hear that you need your medication right now; however, our policy asks that you give us 24 hours. I can compromise and get it to you before the end of the day; however, I am unable to give it to you at this moment.

BE CLEAR ABOUT YOUR ASK

In heated conversations, we often only state facts without acknowledging what we actually need, or we ask for something different from what we actually want. Sometimes we are not even sure what we are asking for until we do not get it. Always know exactly what you are asking for when you need to ask for something; this way, you can be very clear about what it is you need from the other person. I use the example of a roommate arguing over dishes (Many of us have had some form of this argument). One roommate is mad at the other because they never do the dishes, so the difficulty of the tasks falls on them. The roommate who doesn't fulfill their weight does the dishes, but the one who brought up the conversation is still mad, because they did not need the dishes done; they needed to be seen for the hard work they put into the task. Now, everyone is mad because no one feels seen. Slowing down and noticing what you are truly asking for can be a great way to communicate more effectively. *Just recently, I was working with insurance companies as my checks were being sent to an incorrect address. I was transferred to countless people, only to be told to speak to someone else. I continued to ask for my address to be changed and could not find the correct person to talk to. I was getting angry and feeling stuck in the conversations. I finally paused and noticed what I needed in this situation. I need my checks sent to the correct address, but what I needed from the person I was talking to was to find out who I needed to speak with. Eventually, I found the correct contact by asking who I needed to talk with to ensure my checks were sent to the correct place. The issue was resolved. Logically, it seems like they should know that I want to talk to someone who can correct my issue since that is what I was calling about, but I never directly asked for that. When I slowed down and recognized I needed to directly ask for what I needed, I got closer to my goal.*

What exactly do you need when you are asking for something? Once you know exactly what you are asking for, make sure to give many details about the situation.

EXERCISE 18.3 | Clarify what you are asking for

---

1. Notice that you are looping around in the conversation and do not feel heard in what you are asking for. Ask to take a break, "Let me go check into this one second." With practice, you will be able to do this without taking a break, but allow yourself the moment if you need it.

2. Ask what is happening here. Try not to use emotions as you describe this. Using only facts that no one can argue with allows you to communicate more effectively when discussing the topic with the person.

3. Ask yourself what you really need from the person in this situation.

4. Ask again. What do I really need? This might be the same answer, but sometimes you recognize something you were not aware of before.

5. Reflect on the details around the situation that make the ask important.

6. Ask how the ask can be mutually beneficial.

Example: *"I can see that you are very upset about finances. I get that money can be very frustrating. However, you are yelling at me right now, and it is difficult for me to explain my expertise in the situation when emotions are this high.* (Explaining in detail why you are asking can be helpful, as it provides clarity. Yes, it may feel obvious, but it may just need to be said.) *Can you please lower your voice so that we can discuss your concerns? I think it will help us get on the same page."*

Notice how this person asks for exactly what they need. It is tempting to ask them to listen, but the person realizes that what they need first is for them to lower their voice. They point out the facts with validation and why it is getting in the way (because it is difficult for me to explain). They also pointed out how it can be mutually beneficial if they lower their voice because it allows them to be on the same page. This points out that it is not only about me, it is about both of us.

KNOW WHEN TO STEP OUT

If you utilize the above skills for managing your emotions, the next step may be to remove yourself from this situation so that the emotions can calm down. You can do that by making an excuse, "let me look into some other options, I will be right back," or very clearly, because of the person's reactions, "I can see you are very upset, and it is difficult to calm your emotions. I am not sure either of us can be heard in this moment. I am going to step out and will be back in just a moment." This depends on your own personal preference as well as the way that you read the situation in the moment. You may also be required to abide by the rules of your individual clinic.

The argument I hear when I mention this is almost always regarding time. I know that clinics are often crunched for time, because that's part of the job. I know that if you did this in every single appointment, your customer service would eventually be lacking. The hope is that you will use this less often. If you step out for 5 minutes and come back, see if it truly backs up your day, or if the next person is okay with just a few minutes of waiting. If you step out for 5 minutes and spend the whole time feeding your emotions with thoughts like "I can't believe this person sucks this much," you probably aren't going to go back in the room in a better place. Spend the 5 minutes distracting. You can only think one thing at a time (thoughts are likely to bounce quickly in these high-stress moments, but you can really only think one thing at a time). Fill your brain space with a quick game of Tetris, or a task you need to complete that takes brain power and fewer emotions. You can also concentrate on some of the skills in the book that speak to you most. Make sure you set a timer for 5 minutes. It can be easy to forget about the person in the room waiting for you.

When you come back in, ask the person if they are ready to continue. Providing them with the option can help defuse their emotions. If the emotions are just as high on the other end (hopefully they are not for you, that is why you stepped out), give details about the facts, give your professional opinion, and allow them to make the choice that is best for them. Easy right? If they do not allow you to speak, mistreat you, or refuse, it is okay to say, "I have given you the information I have and my professional opinion; this is all I can do for you at this moment." The hope was that they would eventually leave after this interaction. If they do not, it may be time to ask them to leave. If you are worried about a bad review, and this keeps you in these communication patterns, I encourage you to jump to that section of the book.

If you can find composure after you step out, you may be out of your window. You can do some skills naturally that help bring down your emotions. The emergency skills (Exercise 10.1–10.5 and 12.1–12.8) can be great ways to get into your window of tolerance.

Veterinarian: These recurring ear infections may be due to an allergy. We can run an allergy test to determine exactly what he is allergic to, or we can consider adjusting his diet. This is definitely a dog who needs his ears cleaned often. We can discuss this as well.

Handler: That is the stupidest thing I have ever heard. You guys are always trying to get another penny from me. How much profit do you make from that food company when you recommend it? Plus, he doesn't like his ears cleaned. This is where both your nervous systems are changing. You may become defensive about best practice, while the handler becomes defensive about time and money.

The veterinarian in this case may read their own spontaneous body language. Her arm muscles are tight, and her jaw begins to clench. She is having thoughts about how hard she has worked for this information, how dare this person? If they only knew my money struggles? Etc. She now takes a large exhale and starts to guess the handler's nervous system. He is scared of the financial constraints. He worries about his dog. He is angry based on these fears. The veterinarian is now allowed to exhale and validate the handler, allowing space for the conversation to become productive instead of escalating.

Veterinarian: "I understand that the price of things can get frustrating, and time is a constraint. These veterinary visits can be very frustrating, I know. Unfortunately, we are unable to alter the cost; however, we can discuss a mutual agreement based on the options available to both of us. The food change would be less costly than the allergy test, if that helps in your decision. I am happy to show you how to clean the ears quickly so that you do not have to come back here with ear infections so often, and maybe can save yourself some time. Would that help?"

Do you notice how the veterinarian in this example validates where the customer is coming from, asks for what they need as well, and asks them about a solution, given the facts, allowing for a reciprocal conversation? They feel included instead of talked to in the conversation. Hopefully, in this case, the person will begin to communicate options that make sense for the animal. They may still leave the clinic frustrated that they have to spend more time and money than expected on their pet, and this is a valid emotion. Sometimes, news is just frustrating, but with effective communication, they are less likely to take it out on you and are more likely to leave with whatever works best for them.

TALKING TO EACH OTHER

One of the things I've noticed about veterinary clinics is that when emotions run high, people often struggle to communicate effectively with one another. Since emotions are often high, sometimes interactions as a team can be strained (or in worse cases, toxic). Within the natural reaction of stress, people's voice tone naturally becomes more directive, sharper, and louder. Imagine speaking softly with some fluffy fillers in a life-or-death situation. It doesn't work. You need people to know what to do and how to do it quickly. When the clinic gets emergent and rushed, the body changes to an emergency response spontaneously. When we are not actually in a life-or-death situation, people interpret this as anger and bitchiness. They may become defensive as well, and there goes the culture of the clinic. This is part of the reason noticing your nervous system responses is so incredibly important to keeping a culture of well-being.

It is important to notice when your nervous system is in an emergent, frantic state and if it is actually necessary, given the circumstances. If it is necessary at that moment, a repair or check-in may be needed after everything settles. If it is not necessary, you may need to be especially aware of your tone and reactions until you can find the moment you need to relax your nervous system and take a deep exhale before barking orders. A repair may still be needed, depending on how you reacted before checking in.

The same skills we use to communicate with handlers effectively are also effective in communicating with each other. Validation, detailed asks, and knowing your own nervous system are just as important when we talk to each other, especially in difficult conversations or conversations where we check in on each other's well-being.

If you may have offended someone, take a moment to check in with them.

AFTER THE CONVERSATION

When a difficult conversation is over, it can be tempting to ruminate about the audacity of the other person and the way that they treated you. This is the body's way of validating itself. However, it can create complexity in future conversations throughout the day. You may become so agitated by this one person that you become irritable with other undeserving individuals. Your body system may perceive everything that is said to you as aggressive because it is on guard, waiting to fight others who cross your boundaries. If you find yourself so agitated that it is difficult to go on with your day in the best way possible, I recommend this exercise.

EXERCISE 18.4 Pushing on a wall

When you get stuck ruminating about an interaction that made you mad, it is because you cannot complete the emotional cycle. It is stuck fighting the sabretooth tiger without being able to find safety. This exercise activates the muscles that would be needed in a true emergency, telling the brain that it is safe to complete the cycle.

1. Find a wall with clear space to push against.

2. Set yourself up in a plank-type position on the wall.

3. Push as hard as you can on the wall as if you are trying to move the wall.

4. Begin to pedal your feet while pushing against the wall.

5. Do this for 20–40 seconds.

6. Stand back from the wall and see if you notice anything.

EXERCISE 18.5 Tightening and releasing muscles

This is also helpful if you get stuck in an anger responds and just can't get out. The exercise activates muscles in your body as if you are fighting, allowing the body to realize you worked toward fighting danger, and the threat is no longer present.

1. Notice your breath as it is naturally right now. See you if you make it deeper and longer without making the symptoms worse. (If you cannot, no worries, just move on with the most comfortable breath)

2. Tighten all of the muscles in your body. Clench your fist, shrug your shoulders, bring your feet up to tighten your legs, curl your toes, pull your abs in, scrunch your face, tighten your buttocks. True to tighten as much as you possibly can. (If you have an injury or this hurts a part of your body, skip it.)

3. Take a few breaths in the tighten position.

4. With a long, deep exhale, release all of the tension in your body and allow your body to relax as if it were a rag doll

5. Do this exercise two or three times if needed.

EXERCISE 18.6 Repair after a difficult conversation

If you reflect on the interaction and realize you did not communicate effectively, a repair may be in order. This can be true for handlers, each other, or loved ones. It can be difficult to bring up a difficult conversation, but following through with a repair can be essential in maintaining a positive relationship.

Here are the steps for a repair:

1. Check in with the person and see how they are doing after the interaction. *Hey, how are you doing? Things were a little stressful earlier.*

2. Own that you messed up and did not communicate effectively under stress. *I definitely let*

that moment get the best of me and did not treat you the way I would hope to treat someone I care about.

3. Acknowledge ways in which you will work on changing your behavior to be kinder. Ensure you make every effort to implement these changes effectively. *I am going to try to start catching myself and breathing before I get to that point in the future.*

4. Ask if they need anything more. *Is there anything else I can do to make you feel more comfortable? I know it's not easy to be yelled at.*

5. Allow them time to be mad at you. They are still allowed to be mad even if you apologize. The apology makes it easier for them to move past the mad.

Open, effective communication in repairs not only allows space for people to make mistakes without being judged, but it also keeps this person from retaliating with the next person they communicate with. You can break the cycle of high-stress communication with a quick repair. Sometimes we do not realize we acted out of line until our car ride home, when we review our day. It is okay to pull the person aside the next day and repair. It is never too late to make the repair. Maybe they say, "You're good, I get it, I was over it before we left last night." Great, you don't have to continue, but still follow through with the ways in which you plan to make changes.

TALKING TO STAFF WHO MAY BE STRUGGLING

Professionals often ask me, what do I do when someone else is out of their window in the clinic. Depending on the culture of your clinic and the hierarchy, it may be beneficial to talk with that person. Becoming more irritable is a sign of compassion fatigue, burnout out and vicarious trauma. It can be very helpful to discuss this from a place of concern. If it is appropriate to talk about some of the concepts in this book within the clinic, it is helpful so that the language can be the same among all staff. If that is not the culture you are working in, that is okay. Validate the person's stress and encourage them to take a moment to relax outside. Example: *Hey, you seem like today is a little hard, let me cover some of your stuff for 10 minutes so you can step outside and take a breath, or a bite, or whatever you need.* Hopefully, this will lead by example and allow you the space to do the same. If it is more than just a moment, here is an example of a conversation you can have.

SAM: *"Hey, Kim can we talk?"*
       "This job can be very hard for many reasons, and the difficulty can sneak up on you. I noticed that you have been quicker to snap at some of the techs and moving a little slower between appointments. I am concerned that things may be difficult for you right now. Is everything okay?" (Notice the validation and clear facts used.)

KIM: *"I am fine."*

SAM: *"I know this can be difficult to talk about, and I need you to speak more kindly to people around you. What can I do to support you* in this process?" (Notice how I used "and" instead of "but". It tends to solidify the importance of certain situations. Also, notice the importance of asking questions that make the person an active part in the conversation. It is much more comfortable to work with someone than to be talked at.)

KIM: *"I am fine, I will try harder."*

SAM: *"Thank you, I appreciate that. It can be very hard and sometimes impossible to simply try harder in this high-stress environment. I would love to help you manage some of this stress to make trying harder just a little easier."*

KIM: *"I am just so sick of people not taking me seriously. I went to tons of schools, and I am a good veterinarian. Why does everyone question that?"*

SAM: *"This can be very difficult, and I think every veterinarian has felt that way in one moment or another. What can the clinic do to support you?"* (So much validation)

KIM: *"I don't think I have a place here, honestly. I am not sure if I want to be anywhere."*

SAM: *"Do you want to kill yourself?"* (Notice the clarity and directness of this question.)

KIM: *"No, I haven't gotten there yet. I just don't feel like I fit in anywhere."*

SAM: *"Can I get you some resources that help veterinarians get through the blips in the field? I think it would be helpful for you to feel better."*

KIM: *"Yeah, that's fine."*

SAM: *"In the meantime, what can I do to help you here at the clinic? I want to support you and allow for open communication, I also need to ensure that our Vet techs are treated well."* (Continuing to remind the person why you are bringing this up, in a kind way, can be helpful to reiterate it is not just for them. Those who are more team-oriented may be more likely to work on themselves if it is for others more than themselves.)

KIM: *"I can see that. I don't know?"*

SAM: *"What if we work together to reset throughout the day. Would you be okay to join a goal of mine to exhale more throughout the day? I do it when I pass the back door. I think it will allow you to be a little naturally calmer."* (Acknowledging something that works for you and joining as a team can feel less intimidating.)

VALUES AND COMMUNICATION

When we speak from two different value systems, it sounds like we are speaking two different languages. Understanding someone else's value systems and how they are similar to or different from your own can facilitate acceptance of another person, foster connection with people who are different from ourselves, and enhance overall communication with both those we like and those we do not. This does not mean you have to know every detail of the values, but high-level value beliefs are often obvious. Let's say mental well-being and self-exploration are one of the primary values you listed. You are asking for a team meeting where mindfulness is incorporated. The influential people in your clinic have a value of efficiency use of time and do not understand that mindfulness can, in fact, make the clinic more efficient. You ask about mindfulness workshops, and they brush you off, speaking about how it will get in the way of the workload. You realize that efficiency is more important to them than their well-being. You may ask for mindfulness by listing ways in which mindfulness increases efficiency in a workplace. They may still decline a team meeting, including mindfulness, stating that team meetings cannot be billed and are therefore not efficient. However, addressing the issue based on the other person's value system allows more space for you to be heard differently. Perhaps you can find additional research on the topic of mindfulness and efficiency, and suggest that staff members could benefit from learning from a mindfulness expert outside of regular working hours. Eventually, they agree to give you an hour after hours for a mindfulness workshop. If you speak in your language, they may never understand what is needed. They may see it as a waste of time. Speaking from the other person's values allows you to be heard even when you disagree with them.

Knowing the other person's values may also help when you are not feeling heard, no matter how hard you are using your skills. Sometimes our values are so misaligned that it is difficult ever to see where the other is coming from. No matter how much we work, we are in two different worlds, speaking two different languages. Knowing this from a value perspective (knowing both yours and their values) allows space for us to accept the situation as it is. It can protect us from feeling like it is a personal attack and will enable us to acknowledge when we are just different.

EXERCISE 18.7 Values in communication

1. Think about someone you do not get along with. This can be personal or professional.

2. Think of one thing that you butt heads about.

3. Guess what the value is that the other person holds that clashes with yours.

4. Recognize that you probably feel like you are right and they are wrong based on values. In the same way, they feel like they are right and you are wrong.

5. Try to view this person from a slightly different perspective.

6. Write a script discussing the conflict with the person using their values.

Here is a personal example:

My daughter plays soccer. There is a parent on her team that we have encountered over several years of life in various settings. She always rubbed me the wrong way. As I sat on the sidelines listening to her scream for her child and asking everyone to pass to her child, I would cringe. I would leave the field feeling like I ran a marathon; my muscles were so tight. At some point in the season, I realized this person is not going anywhere. She will continue to show up in my life and the life of my child. I asked myself, I wonder what is happening here. I was able to identify that she holds the value that her job as a parent is to help her child succeed. She wants the best for her child, and she believes that the way to do this is by building her up in this way. She likely holds a value that is more individualized. I hold a very strong value of community. In this situation, that means wanting the whole team to succeed. I get genuinely excited when the shy player scores a goal, or the girls do a play that works together as a team. I acknowledge that I feel like I am right, and if you hold a similar value to my own, you may too, but the reality is we are both trying to do the best thing for our child and model

what we believe is the best lesson for our child. She is still not my favorite to sit next to during a soccer game, but I can now see her in a new light. I can tolerate her when she shows up in my life time and time again. I can be friendlier with her. Most importantly, I can sit through a game without my muscles tightening in a defensive manner, ready to fight off a bear. I will never agree with her, and I doubt we will ever be close friends (although you never know), but now I can tolerate her, and I leave feeling better.

Here is how I used this skill in a conversation at work:

I used to work for an agency with very strict rules about time in the office. They were not flexible with adjusting hours in any way at all. I was contemplating moving jobs as my learning in that position had stalled. I was part of a specialized group there that I enjoyed and which helped me grow and thrive; however, all other aspects of the job conflicted with a value of mine that includes continued learning and growth. I talked with my boss about potentially moving to part-time and only working in the specialized program. I presented him with benefits that would serve the team as a whole and the company's mission. I explained how I could save the company money because they would no longer be paying my benefits, and I would use whatever empty office space I could find, so they would not have to supply a full-time office (I knew that money and space were strong values of the company). I fully expected my boss to say no, and I would have to prepare for leaving the entire company. When I presented this opportunity from his perspective, I was approved as a part-time employee. I know other people who were denied this opportunity because they presented the opportunity from their own values of quality care and fairness. I fully believe talking to them from their point of view is the only thing that gave me that opportunity.

PREPARING AND DECOMPRESSING FROM A DIFFICULT INTERACTION

It can be helpful to prepare when you know you are going into a difficult interaction. Just because you prepare does not mean that you have to say exactly what you prepared to say. In fact, you probably won't, but going through these steps makes it more likely you will use the skills you need to be as effective as you can in the conversation. Remember, each reaction and interaction is a learned experience. You can use it to build resilience for the next difficult conversation that you have. In Figure 18.1, you can see a breakdown of what this may look like using the exercises discussed.

Sometimes you do not have time to prepare. The conversation happens fast, and you use the skills to the best of your ability. In this case, it is effective to review the conversation when you are done. I know it can feel like you do not have time for that. However, if you spend a few minutes on this when you get home, it can help build brain pathways, making it more likely for you to use the skills the next time a difficult conversation arises. If you are spending time ruminating about the conversation anyway, doing it in a more organized way can allow you to feel more settled so you can move on with your day or evening. Figure 18.2 shows a flowchart you can follow, allowing you to ask, "What did I do well?" and "What did I miss?" in that conversation.

PRACTICE MAKES PERMANENT

By reading this section of this book, I do not think the next time you have a difficult situation at work, you are magically going to come up with an amazing communication style. I wish it were that easy. The thing is, the more you practice these concepts, the better you will be at them. Here we are again, needing more time that just may not exist. A good way to practice this is after an interaction that you don't feel went well. Going through these steps afterwards and deciding how you would have handled it with more practice actually builds the neuropathways for the next time, so that you can do better in the future. It allows you to learn from your mistakes. You can do this

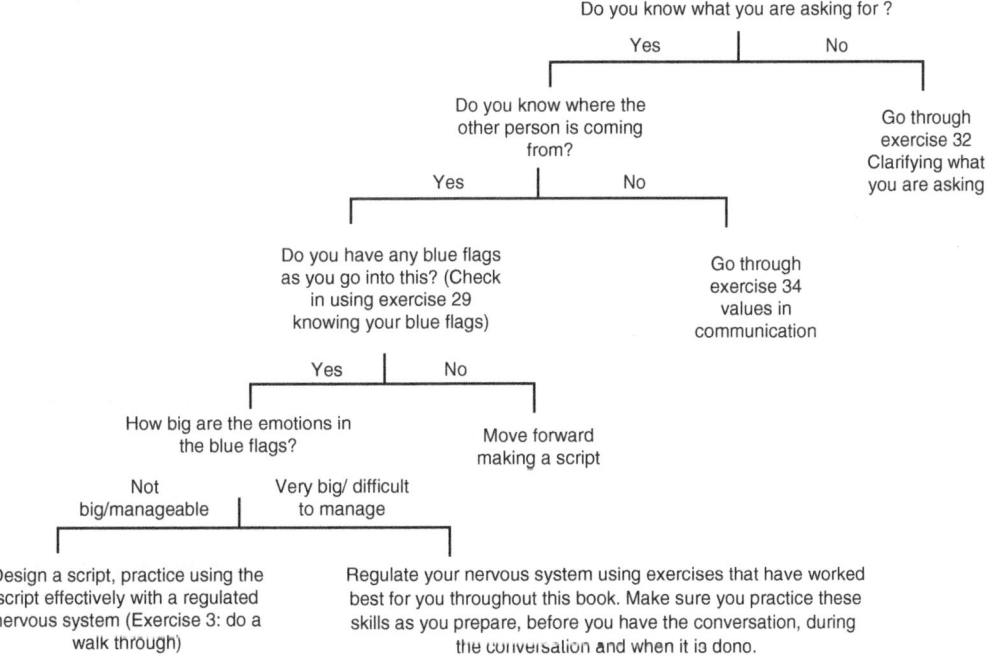

FIGURE 18.1   A flowchart showing steps for preparing for a difficult conversation.

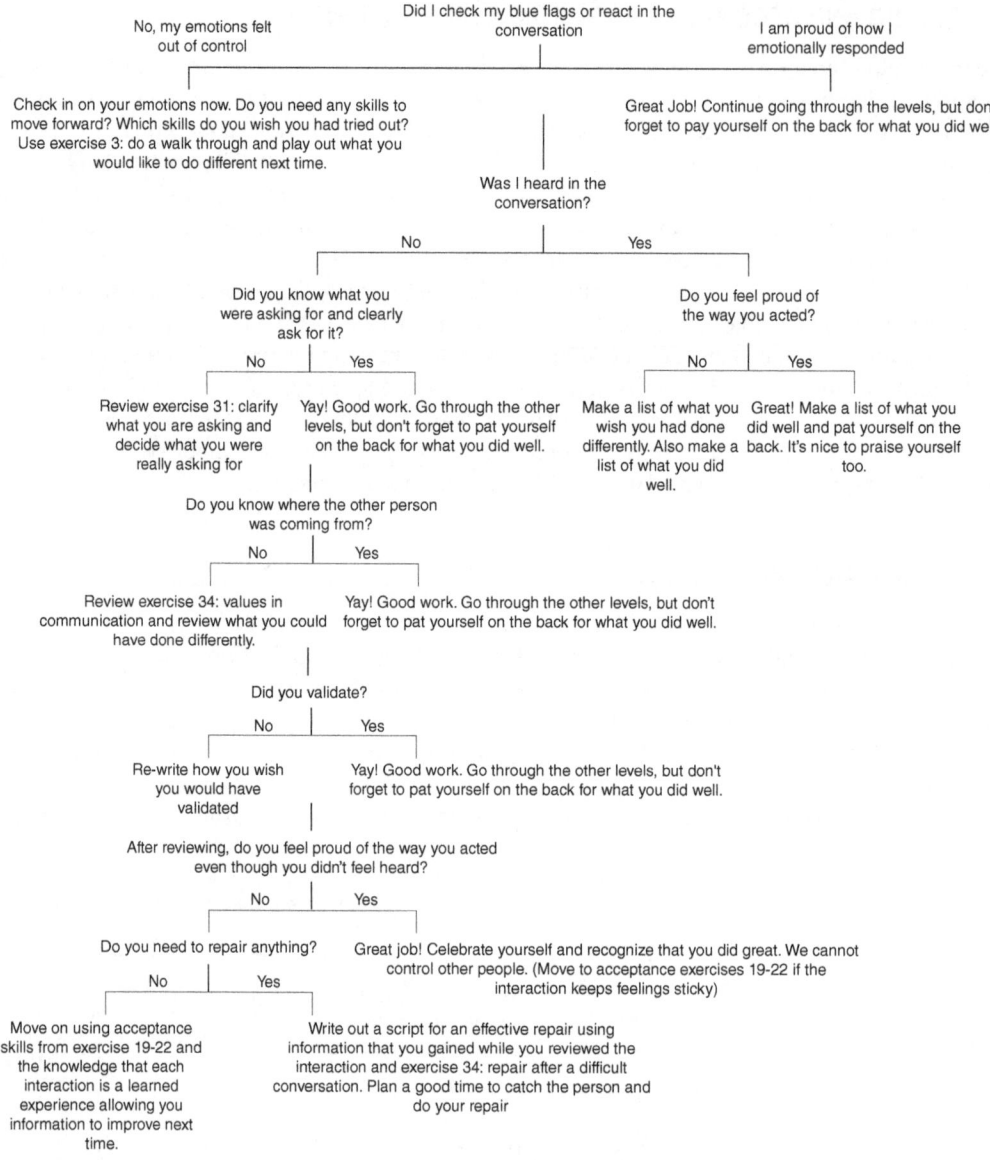

FIGURE 18.2 A flowchart to follow when assessing effectiveness after a difficult conversation.

during your commute or while doing something else. Be careful not to be critical of yourself and hold all the things you can do differently. This is about curiosity, learning, and finding ways to grow.

Another way to practice is right before a difficult conversation. If you know you are planning on having a hard conversation with a colleague, superior, or loved one, look through the steps for effective communication. Write out what you could say in a clear way that is validating. Practice what you would say and how you would say it. Ground yourself and have the conversation. You may not say exactly what you wrote out and practiced. In fact, you probably won't. However, you are more likely to have all the components and communicate more effectively just by writing it out and thinking about what and how you will say the hard thing.

I know that the example communications can sound clunky and unrealistic. I give the perfect, textbook example of the way communication can look. It may look different when you actually do it. It likely won't be perfect, as the examples show. It may also be clunky because you haven't practiced this form of communication as much. It is okay for it to be different, and it is okay for it to be clunky. The important thing to keep in mind is that if you hold these components in communication, you are more likely to have effective communication. The more you practice, the more fluid the skills will become, taking out the clunky and different that may get in the way of effective communication right now.

FOOD FOR THOUGHT JOURNAL TOPIC:

1. What is communication like for you with your colleagues, handlers, family, and friends?

2. Where do you feel like you communicate very well, given the skills discussed?

3. Where do you feel like you could improve your communication skills and how?

4. What feels scary about applying these skills? (This one is likely more of the free-flow journaling style.)

REFERENCE

Stetina, B. U. and Krouzecky, C. (2022). 'Reviewing a decade of change for veterinarians: Past, present and gaps in researching stress, coping and mental health risks', *Animals*, 12(22), 3199. https://doi.org/10.3390/ani12223199.

CHAPTER 19

Expectations

Expectations come from all directions: expectations of yourself, expectations from clients, and expectations from the people we work for. Expectations are not always a bad thing. They can serve as an unspoken manual for the way we can behave and practice well. The problem lies when the expectations are unrealistic. Unrealistic expectations are significant causes of imposter syndrome, burnout, and other work-related stressors, making it unsafe to disappoint people around you, make mistakes, or admit to not knowing something. Veterinarians constantly juggle expectations and obligations to peers, society, themselves, their employer, and sometimes future employers. Many times this is complicated by conflicting expectations, making it inevitable that someone will be disappointed (Stretiva). Most of us are unaware of the expectations we hold within our bodies, especially those we hold for ourselves. They hidden barriers getting in the way of being the most effective person we can be.

EXPECTATIONS FROM HANDLERS

People come to a veterinary clinic with the hope that they will be able to "fix" their animal or at least keep them healthy. This is a reasonable expectation on paper, but when it comes to a complicated case or a terminal animal, this can become an unrealistic expectation. This is complicated by technology that has made it more likely for you to help an animal in need, while also making it more expensive at the same time. While your primary allegiance is to the practice of animal health, at some point, there is a level of customer service that can sometimes border on people-pleasing. It can feel unsafe not to please a handler, from a nervous system perspective. Maybe you are scared of the negative review. Perhaps you have been yelled at or accosted by enough people that not pleasing a client means you will be verbally and emotionally attacked. This may also be related to a belief system that you are responsible for others' emotions. This belief system can stem from behaviors exhibited by adults in your earlier life, messages conveyed to you blatantly or covertly, or simply the way you were born. It can also be a mixture of all of the above or something else.

Contrasting with the people-pleasing response to expectations, some people have the opposite response to this. They do not care about the expectations of handlers at all. This can stem from compassion fatigue, a belief system that the veterinarian is always right, or messages you received throughout your life. While this may be regarded as a correct response by some, it also overlooks the patient's needs and the customer service aspect of the job.

Like most things in life, the answer lies somewhere in between the two extremes. The human body tends to pendulate between extremes when neither extreme works. We go from "Oh my gosh, I can't believe I upset that person so much," to "F'em all, no one cares about what I have to say, so why should I care what they have to say." Compassion and understanding of others are very important in relationships, which, like it or not, is part of the job.

I wish I could require everyone in the world to be nice, and I wish I could educate everyone about realistic expectations, but I can't. People perceive you as an expert and therefore have high expectations of you. While I can't change the high expectations, my goal is to help you manage how you deal with them.

A first step in addressing the responsibility to meet all expectations of handlers is to recognize when you are feeling guilty, overly pleasing, disconnected, or any other reaction that indicates you are struggling with expectations.

You are allowed to feel guilt. It is designed to help you adhere to your own values and those of the larger society. However, it can often be unjustified when addressing expectations. When an emotion does not fit the facts of the situation, an effective coping strategy is to do the opposite of what the emotion is telling you to do. This is a form of exposure because when an emotion is unjustified, it is often because of a subconscious fear of a different emotion. Doing the opposite and surviving allows your body to recognize that the emotion may be safe, contrary to the previous belief. Making a decision and standing by it, even when the client is disappointed, is a form of this exposure. It can be tempting in this situation to feel extreme guilt and think of all the things that you feel guilty about in your life. It is also tempting to avoid guilt by giving the handler what they want. However, neither of these is effective. You get to decide whether the guilt is justified (telling you that you are doing something outside of your morals and values) or if it is unjustified and you need to acknowledge it and move on, allowing it to be.

Sometimes we assume people know what expectations we can meet and which ones we cannot meet. However, you may need to clearly communicate what expectations you can meet versus which ones cannot be met when discussing next steps with a client. The steps listed above can help you do this more effectively.

EXERCISE 19.1	Managing expectations of handlers

Notice you are falling into a pattern related to expectations from handlers. (These could include feelings of anger, sadness because you disagree with someone, imposter syndrome because someone questioned you, or something that is a personal reaction to you.)

1. Ask yourself, where are they coming from?
   Maybe they are a Google search doctor who found false information that needs to be addressed. Maybe they are very stressed that an important animal in their life may be unwell. Maybe they are desperate to save a pet that may not be able to be saved. Maybe they are stressed about finances and feeling annoyed by the additional burden. Take a moment and think about where they might be coming from. *You do not have to agree with the person*. This is a very important component of this. Just because we see where they are coming from does not mean we agree with it.

2. Ask yourself, what is their expectation of me based on where they are coming from?

3. Then ask, is that expectation a reasonable request given the current circumstances?

4. Remind yourself, GUILT WILL NOT HURT YOU. You can feel guilt, it can be unjustified, AND you can do whatever you feel guilty about.

5. Accept the guilt and the logical choice and follow through. (This becomes exposure to guilt, which can naturally decrease it if you feel guilty about feeling guilty).

At first, you may not be able to apply these skills in the given moment. You may have to do this after work, when thinking about the situation before bed, in the car, or wherever you tend to ruminate about the day. It may take a few minutes when you initially do it, because you may need to think about all the steps, pretty hard to find an answer. You may even need to write it out. However, over time, you will learn how to do these steps in moments while talking to a patient. This is a skill that takes practice before it becomes easy for some.

FOOD FOR THOUGHT JOURNALING:

1. What expectations do handlers have of me?

2. What expectations are reasonable, which are not?

3. Where do I avoid guilt in my life?

4. What steps can I take to practice feeling guilty and tolerating it while still maintaining my standards and expectations?

EXPECTATIONS OF OTHERS IN THE FIELD

The one thing I notice about veterinarians is that they are just as hard on each other as they are on themselves. This comes from the high standards of the field itself and is learned in graduate school. The culture is one of high achievement. You learn that being hard on each other can help each other grow. This is a true strength of the profession in some ways. However, it does not allow much space for fallibility. Standards of care regarding legal and ethical standards are very high in the field. This is necessary for the integrity of veterinary medicine; however, it also increases the stress of those practicing on a day-to-day basis. I encourage you to notice where professional expectations are serving a much-needed purpose and where they are unachievable. Try to focus on achievable expectations instead of those that can't be met. When the ones that can't be met are the focus, it can be debilitating.

Sometimes, people around you may be judging you and holding you to a high standard. At other times, expectations from others in the field are more perceived than real. This is because we all want to be the best we can be. We feel like everyone is watching and judging because we are watching and judging ourselves. However, this also means that if anyone sees our weakness (a mistake we made due to not knowing all the information), we could be brought to our knees. Vulnerability is a great way to treat expectations when they are perceived. I recommend openly discussing fallibility with the safest people. This can be exceptionally challenging at first because it requires us to be vulnerable. Still, it can open up a conversation of fallibility, hopefully creating a trickle effect where others address their fallibility as well. This can be easier said than done, I understand that, so starting small may be a first step. "*Gosh, I don't know the answer to that*" is a form of vulnerability. Also, make sure the person you are trying this with is safe. If you pick a person who is generally pretty hard on you, you will prove yourself right.

Sometimes you are the one holding expectations of others. Recognize that while expectations are important, it is also important to give each other grace. This is a hard field to work in. Each person in the clinic holds a challenging job. Check in on your expectations of others. When you notice yourself holding unrealistic expectations of others, start to notice the person's strengths and how they can be helpful to you in the long run. Start expressing gratitude for these strengths out loud to people around you. Consider what others do well and compliment them on their strengths. Everyone has a strength and is needed in the clinic for it to function smoothly, creating a peaceful environment as a veterinary clinic can. When this is acknowledged, it can positively change the vibe of the clinic. You will also notice an increase in efficiency and effectiveness. People work better with confidence.

When a superior holds expectations of you that you cannot meet, it is important to recognize what this expectation is. Being able to define the expectation in words may allow you to fact-check whether this expectation is reachable and create steps to try to achieve it. When you fact-check, you may not fully understand the expectations that have been given to you. If you cannot put the expectation into words, it can be important to ask the person what their expectation of you is. This can be extremely terrifying, but I hope that through open conversation, we can clarify what the person's expectation is and what you perceive it to be. With open communication, we can also discuss tangible steps the person recommends we take to start meeting these expectations. We also know what we are working for, which feels more grounded than just guessing. When we slow down and clearly label our expectations, we start to understand each other better and work together more effectively. If the person continues to be unreasonable, this exposes a need to change workplaces to a more supportive environment.

EXPECTATION OF OURSELVES

We can be our own worst critics, that is for sure. Veterinarians are categorized as high achievers. This has many strengths to it. High achievers often possess a significant amount of drive, determination, and the ability to challenge themselves and grow. However, this also comes with a desire to be overly hard on ourselves for our flaws. With every strength comes a flaw, and with every flaw comes a strength. It is far easier to concentrate on the flaws because it feels as if we can recognize our shortcomings, and we can fix them. The reality is that we begin to fight them for the rest of our lives and often feel pretty crummy about ourselves along the way. If we were only to concentrate on our strengths, we may not see our flaws and have a hard time working with them in a way that they interfere less. When we focus on our strengths just as much as our flaws, the strengths shine, while we learn to work with the flaws. We can create realistic expectations of ourselves. Most people notice their flaws way more than their strengths. For this reason, I encourage you to overcompensate and spend extra time on your areas of strength. If a skier is trying to avoid a tree, they look toward the clear slope ahead of them. If they look at the tree while telling their body not to run into the tree, the body will turn and run into the tree. If they do not notice the tree at all, they may lose concentration and run into it. When they acknowledge the tree is there and decide to focus on the clear path ahead, they will likely get down the mountain safely. If you are someone who never acknowledges your flaws, you may have to spend more time thinking about what you can do better. As Figure 19.1 shows, it is easy to concentrate on either all of your strengths ignoring your flaws, or all of your flaws ignoring your strengths, but real clarify comes when you notice strengths and flaws equally. You are able to see where you can utilize the strength and where you can find help with your flaws. You no longer have to fix anything you can simply see the best way for you to succeed.

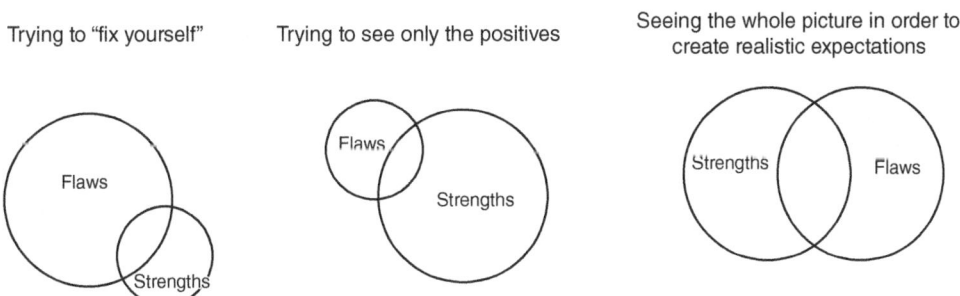

FIGURE 19.1   Circles are drawn to show the drawback to concentrating more on strengths and flaws in relation to the benefit of noticing equal parts strengths and flaws.

The first step in addressing high expectations of yourself is to stop shoulding on yourself. When I was a young therapist, I gave a talk to a group of people of all ages about behavioral changes. There was an elderly couple in the group, and both were hard of hearing. I spoke to the group about the danger of should and stated, "You shouldn't, should on yourself." To which the women shouted, "What?" and the man shouted, "Don't poop on yourself."

While he did not hear me correctly, he was saying the same thing I was. When we state the word "Should," it is often great information that we are likely addressing something that is an unrealistic expectation. I should practice better self-care, I should eat better, I should exercise, I should have known that............. All of these shoulds are a sign of being hard on yourself. Shoulds often come from other people's values and not our own, making it hard to internalize and follow through with. Now, yes, there are things that science suggests would create a better lifestyle. Diet and exercise definitely fall into that category, but changing our language from *"I should...." (Being very hard on ourselves)* to *"how am I going to...."* can change the feel of it altogether. If you are not doing the thing you wish you were doing (or should be doing), it is likely because the step you are trying to take is too big. Slow it down and see if a different avenue may work better before you go down the dark hole of shoulds.

Now comes the next part of the saying, "You shouldn't should on yourself." The word should is going to pop into your brain. Here is the point where we can fall into a vicious cycle. *I was told that "should" is a word that I shouldn't use because it is me being mean to myself, and now here I am using it. Gosh, here I am failing again.* NOPE. As you work on your mental well-being and apply the skills in this book, you are not going to be perfect. Instead of berating yourself every time you think the word, SHOULD, maybe just notice that should comes up, so you might be being hard on yourself, and begin to use skills directed at reframing those thoughts. "Should" can become a blue flag, providing you with information for your next steps, rather than a red flag indicating danger.

While "should" is a huge blue flag, another large blue flag is "but". We try to be nice to ourselves and notice our strengths and say something like, "I am very nice to people BUT that leads to people pleasing" or "I have a great attention to detail, BUT I also miss large pieces that could be important." Yes we notice our strengths but we are communicating that they are not as good as the flaw. When you are only noticing your flaws, it becomes habitual to only notice the negative. We start to put blinders on, not much different from blinders you would put on a horse, so that they do not see the distractions in your peripheral vision. Anything that is not in our direct line of vision (flaws, mishaps, and failed expectations) becomes unsafe. When we challenge ourselves to notice small strengths or potential strengths without the "but" and without the "should," we can start to stretch the blinders out until we no longer need them. We begin to see the big picture, both good and bad, which allows for better problem-solving, a clearer path toward growth, and better well-being. I encourage you to use "and" instead of "but."

Let's say you are someone who struggles to find your strengths, and the idea of exploring any strength makes you freeze in your tracks. That is absolutely okay. Start small. Notice some things that are potential strengths and try them on for size. Maybe they fit and maybe they don't. If they don't, no problem, try something else and see how that fits.

I tend to be a very big-picture person. This means that details often escape me. I forget where I left my keys, wallet, and shoes on a regular basis. This is something that I am very hard on myself about. I see others hang their keys up in the same place no matter what, so why can't I establish this pattern? Over time, I began to recognize my gift of being a big-picture person. I can also put two detailed pieces together to form a clearer image without having to learn something new. I continue to struggle with details, but that will not change. I learned to put tracking devices on the things I misplace the most so that I do not waste my time. I also learned to give extra time to find stuff and to set things out if I know I will be crunched for time. When I am not distracted by the negative thoughts, I tend to be less scattered-brained. I allow myself to focus on big pictures and use my strength to the fullest, while asking others to check my details when necessary. I also allow myself more time when I need to concentrate on details in a project. Knowing I have a big-picture mind and embracing this allows me to work backwards from where I once did. I now start with the idea and find details that fit this idea. I am far less likely to miss a detail when it relates to my big-picture strength. I am also less stuck because I am not trying to start with details, as certain people told me I should. My work is more effective, more efficient, and has far fewer mistakes. I also know where to ask for help because I know I am more prone to miss a small detail. I like myself more because I can see both the strengths and weaknesses and where it is tied. It also allows me to see others' strengths and weaknesses because there are many people who struggle to see the big picture as they concentrate on their strength of details. I still get frustrated with myself when things are not where they should be or I miss a detail, but I have learned to live with it in a more effective way.

You likely have expectations of yourself about how you will function after reading this book. You may envision yourself walking into the clinic as a new person with amazing skills that sink into your body through osmosis. It can feel defeating to want to try a skill but forget. It can feel hopeless when using skills becomes extremely challenging. I encourage you to use this information to remind your brain and body "that is an unrealistic expectation" and regroup. Calling out unrealistic expectations and rewriting them from a strength perspective may have to be done a million times before it becomes natural, but it is easier than being so dang hard on yourself.

Some of you reading this are frustrated, think, "expectations of myself are what have gotten me to where I am today." You love the expectations you set for yourself because they give you drive. That is perfectly fine as long as the expectations are achievable.

FOOD FOR THOUGHT JOURNALING:

1. What do you expect from yourself at work? What parts of your expectations are realistic? What parts are not?

2. What are your "shoulds"? What are your "buts"?

3. How have your expectations served you? How have they contributed to distress?

USING EXPECTATIONS FOR GOOD, NOT EVIL

Whether expectations come from our handlers, colleagues, or ourselves, they can be valuable information to help us grow, rather than tearing us down. When we slow down the process of expectations and utilize the skills listed above, we can begin to notice that other people's expectations may provide an opportunity to decide how we would like to grow next. This could be personal or professional. Some people's expectations may not fit our value system at all. It may, in fact, contradict our value system, which would communicate something we are not interested in at all. Let's say I am a small animal veterinarian. I do not specialize in dermatology and often send referrals to a colleague down the street who specializes in small animal dermatology. My patients' handlers often expect me to know all things about everything, and sometimes get frustrated that I send them to a different professional. This expectation they hold can allow me to contemplate "should I become more versed in certain dermatology needs?" Maybe I haven't had the opportunity for this type of learning, and it intrigues me. I have decided that this year's CEs will concentrate on small animal dermatology. I will likely still need to send some referrals because I am not a specialist, but I can address some mild concerns more effectively and feel more confident in myself. The handler's expectations of me pushed me out of my comfort zone to allow me to study something that allows me to be better at my job, and I actually find I enjoy it more than I thought I did. On the other hand, the handlers wish I had more dermatology expertise, but I am actually more interested in small animal orthotics and enhancing my skills in this arena. I do not have the time, money, or energy to do both. I decide to continue addressing the patients' needs through referrals more often than addressing them myself. The expectation of the handler, when slowed down, allowed me to really access my goals and interests so that I can grow in my own personal values, strengths, and interests. It exposed my perception that I need to know all things about everything, and allowed me to question the realistic aspect of this expectation of myself. I am now able to accept the expectations of others with reality vs guilt and desire to avoid disappointed handlers. I will likely still feel guilty, but I now know the guilt is not justified. I am able to remind myself that the guilt is my desire to make them happy, but I have decided that this is the best policy for my practice. When we slow down and notice our expectations, it can expose our own values and interests. We can use the expectation for self-reflection, which can allow for personal growth. There is actually no exact right way to address expectations, but in slowing down and fact-checking, you can see what the next steps need to be for ourselves, not for others. When we become more aware, we naturally slow things down, which allows us to see things more clearly, make better decisions based on the reaction, and ultimately nurture our nervous system.

In noticing, fact-checking, and addressing expectations, we naturally challenge our nervous system. As I mentioned before, the well-being challenges that are associated with expectation are often linked to the fact that fallibility and/or guilt will kill or harm us. We are avoiding these feelings at all costs, setting ourselves up for failure because there will always be expectations. By becoming more aware of expectations and addressing them through the skills discussed in this chapter, we begin to expose ourselves to our deep fear of guilt and fallibility. Guilt and fallibility are both unavoidable, universal human traits. We begin to allow safety in the exposure of these traits, which, over time, allows them to be more accessible, which ultimately allows us to work from a more authentic sense of self.

Decision-Making

CHAPTER 20

CONFLICTING OPINIONS IN DECISION-MAKING

When making decisions, it is extremely difficult to balance the belief systems of the handler with those of the clinic and yourself. Money is a very popular way that ethical dilemmas show up in the workplace. People may put finances above their pets' needs either out of value or obligation. (Dickson, 2023). Some people may even see animals differently from the way you do, which can be very distressing. With the rise of companion animals, there has also been a rise in various belief systems about these animals. Some view them as family members, others as tools to carry out a task, and still others as "just an animal." In the court system, pets are seen as legal property, while the owner may see them as family, and you may have a view somewhere in between. The question arises, "whose values do I turn to when making a difficult decision?" When we have a plan of action for what we will do during difficult times, things can become easier. This does not mean that the plan is not flexible. For all the neurotic, Type A individuals, flexibility may be difficult. For those with a more flexible, less rigid approach, the plan may be challenging. Having a base plan can provide a foundation and basis for decision-making, while allowing flexibility creates space for specific cases that do not fit the base plan. There is no right or wrong answer about who you should turn to first in decision-making. For some, it will be their employer; for others, it will be themselves; for some, it will be the handler. No answer is wrong, except the one that does not fit best with the person making the decision. The key here is to know what is true for you so that you always have a default mode and do not waver based on what someone else said you are supposed to do. If there is a legal response to a decision or an answer that falls within professional ethics, this should always be the default response.

Sometimes decisions are so difficult that you become frozen in the moment. It feels like you are not competent to make the decision, or there is no good answer, so you don't know what to do. Practicing making future decisions can help build confidence in your decision-making abilities. While the following exercise takes a considerable amount of time, which is not always possible in a clinic setting, going through these steps can create space for building confidence and making faster decisions in the future. I encourage you to practice them with situations that you expect to arise to build confidence for the future.

EXERCISE 20.1 Decision-making

Before proceeding with the following exercise, ensure you have answers to the following questions. I encourage you to sit with each question so that you ensure you are answering to yourself, not what should be the answer.

1. Who holds the most authority? Your employers, you, or the handler?

2. What is your primary role as a veterinarian?

3. What are the core values you listed when completing exercise 18?

For those who like to write things out. Here are some steps you can take in this decision:

1. Make a list of all possible choices. Some can be ridiculous; make a list of all of them. (I have you list all, even the ridiculous, because sometimes you add an option that is actually more realistic than you thought.)

2. Circle the ones that are actually feasible.

3. What does the handler think? What do you think? What does your employer think?

4. Write out the pros and cons of all the feasible options (this pro and con list is not about finding out which one has more pros. It is a way to think about the details of each decision in as much detail as possible, while also considering the overall outcome.)

5. Write out or picture how you will manage the cons of each of the scenarios.

6. Picture yourself or write out each scenario, start to finish, and notice how you feel about each outcome.

7. Check in to see if you have an answer to what you should do, even if you do not like the answer.

For those who are more visual, the flowchart in Figure 20.1 allows for some structure in decision-making.

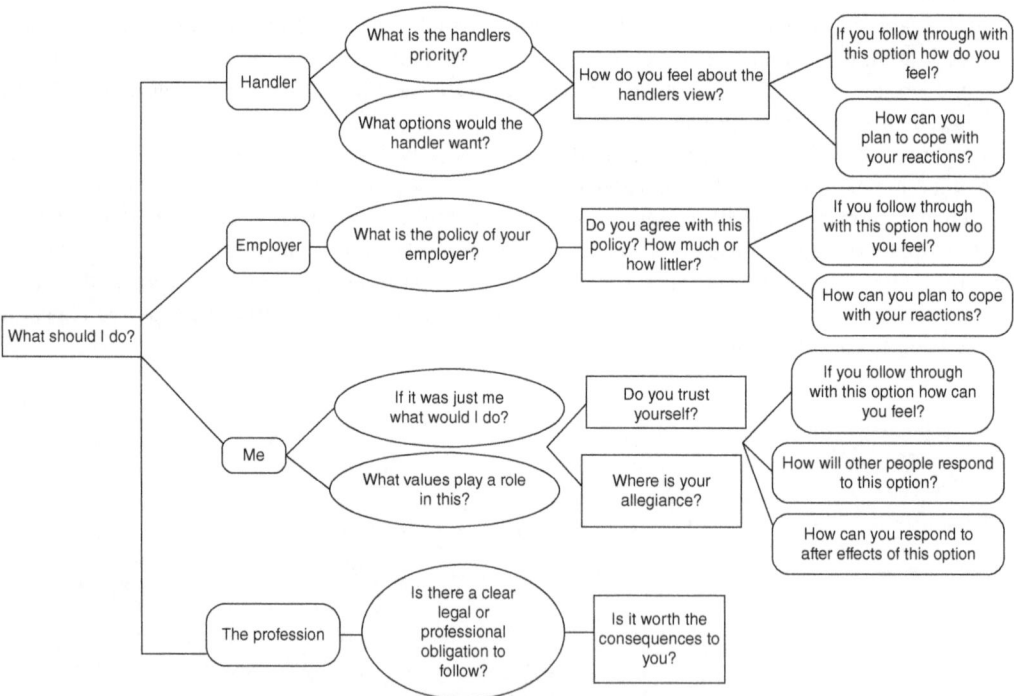

FIGURE 20.1 A flowchart for decision-making that allows for deeper thought processes and more confidence.

WHEN YOU STRUGGLE TO KNOW IF YOU DID THE RIGHT THING

There will be times when you utilize your values and defer to the best decision and still struggle to know if you did the right thing. It is important to know that even when making the best decision, you may still experience imposter syndrome and/or guilt. This does not necessarily mean that you made a bad decision. I believe that we all have a "knower." It is not a fortune teller or an all-knowing part of us, but it is something about us that knows the right answer. This "knower" gets covered up with anxiety and mistrust, so it is hard to find. Let's be clear, it is not always super clear, even when we check in with the "knower." This felt sense allows for a check-in with our body that clears out all the junk associated with it. Yes, this sounds fruity and maybe a little weird. You will likely do this exercise with skepticism (I did the first time I tried it.) It will work for some and not for others. I simply ask that you humor me in this experiment. Some people are very aware of sensations in their bodies and can label them. Some cannot. For some, it is an image or a general felt sense. For some, it is a color or a temperature. Feel free to be creative with this exercise if you would like.

EXERCISE 20.2 | Checking in on your "knower"

---

1. Think of something that you know to be true, no matter what. Something neutral. The color of a wall, or the address of your home. Think about the fact that you know this, no matter what.

2. Do a body scan. For a visual person, this may be picturing a black light going over your whole body, highlighting any tension, tightness, and unusual sensations. For a less visual person, it might be just searching for a sensation. What does knowing feel like? Because this is neutral, it may not be a strong feeling. Some people will be able to locate it in the body? Others will feel like knowing is just knowing. Either is okay; there is still a felt sense that you know. I notice that many people feel this sensation in their torso area.

3. Think of something that you know for a fact is true but that you do not necessarily like. It is not

effective to pick something that has a level 10 of distress; maybe find something that is a 3 or 4. Ideas could be political (again, if it's a lower-level distress), weather-related, or something about a relationship.

4. Check in on where you feel this in your body in a similar way that you did in number 2.

5. You will likely experience different sensations than you did in number 2, but look for some similarities. Maybe your chest still has pressure, or your throat still has an opening. There is no wrong answer here. The answer can be "I just feel like I know."

6. Check in throughout life here and there to see if this is a knowing. Check in with things that are neutral, positive, or negative. Explore what it feels like for this to be a backup in decision-making.

The knowing exercise above suggests that each person actually has a sense of what is right, wrong, and neutral, as it aligns with their life and value system. This knowing gets covered up by anxiety and shoulds. Eventually, we stop trusting it. It becomes hard to differentiate between anxiety and knowing. By doing this exercise, some may be able to discern the difference between the two and begin to find empowerment in decision-making. Others will continue to struggle with trusting or even finding their knowing. If this was ineffective for you, that is perfectly fine. I encourage you to use other skills in this book that you find effective. The purpose of this exercise is to find an anchor that brings you back into your window so that you can make your best decisions. No one skill supersedes another. This is when the best decisions are made.

WHAT IF THERE IS A BAD OUTCOME FROM YOUR DECISION

It can be heartbreaking when the outcome of your decision does not turn out ideal. You can start to question yourself. However, even when the outcome is not ideal, the decision may have been correct. We are the only person we can control. Therefore, the part of our system that would like to find control looks inward and blames itself. These are the times that can lead your brain spinning in a million different directions. The easy response I could give you is "You shouldn't should on yourself." (or Sh*t on yourself, however you prefer it). Which is true, but it only works a tiny little bit, if anything. I could tell you to forgive yourself and move on, but again, that might not be very helpful. I encourage you to do both of these skills, but more importantly, I encourage you to give yourself time to grieve the outcome. I encourage you to make a list of all the things you have learned from this situation.

I encourage you to take a limited amount of time to research more information so you can make a better decision next time. While research and learning more about a topic can help us grow and be more knowledgeable, and is not in itself a bad thing, it can be very tempting to hyper-research a topic in hopes that it will reduce our anxiety. We want to be aware of this. If you are prone to hyper-researching, decide on a time limit. It can be an hour, or a day, or whatever feels reasonable to you. During that time, research as much as you can. Visualize using the new information the next time a situation arises. Remind yourself that it is unclear what would have happened if you had made a different decision. If you knew the answer to the outcome, it would not be a difficult decision.

Don't forget to try to remind your brain that it is not the only case you have had this week. Our brain gets tunnel vision and only focuses on the cases that didn't go perfectly or that we struggled with, causing us to forget the cases that went really well and the decisions that flowed smoothly. It is very likely that both happened in the day, and I am extremely confident that both happened in your week. Our brain communicates a message that if you don't focus on the negative outcomes and crappy parts of your day, you will miss something and ultimately do the most dangerous thing for the animal. However, our brain is missing a huge piece of the puzzle. If you don't notice and spend some time focusing on the cases that went really well, it is more difficult to replicate that in future decision-making. It is important to review positive outcomes to give space to learn from those as well. Each outcome is a learning experience to make us better for future cases. When we view them this way, they become less anxiety-provoking.

EXERCISE 20.3 | Shifting thought patterns

If you are someone who ruminates on things as you leave work and throughout the night. I encourage you to find a routine where you ask yourself these questions as you leave work.

1. Notice you are only noticing the negative, and remind yourself that both positive and negative exist and are important.

2. What did I do well today?

3. What did I learn today from all my experiences, positive and negative (Make sure you review both)?

4. What do I plan to do to be better tomorrow?

5. What do I plan to do to be better when I get home?

When this exercise is not a habit, and you are used to thinking of the negative and difficult, it can be extremely challenging. Allow it to be superficial at first. The cool thing is, when you do this a few times, you really do learn a great deal, which tells the brain that you succeeded in a really positive way, and you will begin to spend a little more time in the positive outcomes. You focus on the hard stuff because you want to be the best you can be. When you learn a path to the best you can be, it is also easier to focus on what went right; it becomes easier and faster. Notice that I do not encourage you to only focus on the positive. Both positive and negative exist in our lives. It is important to make sure we notice both. The reality is that both good and bad are happening, and we are working on opening up the blinders and bringing awareness to all aspects of life.

YOUR NERVOUS SYSTEM AND DECISION-MAKING

At some point, I learned that my body thought making a mistake was just as dangerous as a sabre-tooth tiger. We can blame it on our heritage, the school system, or the judgment of others. The problem is that when you feel unsafe making a decision, it becomes debilitating. When you cannot learn from a decision that did not go the way you wished it would, you cannot gain the information you need to be better and stronger. Not only are you not able to learn from decisions when you are debilitated, but you also start to perceive decisions themselves as unsafe. Even a simple question like, where are we going to get dinner tonight, feels excruciating. The fatigue of decision-making creates some messages within the nervous system that making the wrong decision, no matter how important it is, is dangerous. It sounds weird to think that your body believes that eating tacos when you should have had a hamburger would kill you, but our nervous systems are not very logical. When you add to this the fact that in veterinary medicine, you are sometimes making life-and-death decisions for an animal, the stress increases multifold.

When you can calm your nervous system and build your confidence, you will find that decisions become faster, more effective, and less exhausting.

EXERCISE 20.4   Grounding with something that feels good

1. When you are not under stress, pick 3–5 words or a picture that represents something true about you that you believe. What are you best at? What do people compliment you on? When have you felt the best in your life? Perhaps it is remembering the feeling of summiting a mountain and realizing you are strong, or trying out surfing and feeling proud of your bravery. Maybe it is your graduation gown and crossing the stage, or a hug from someone you love. It could be a message like, "I retain a lot of knowledge," "I am smart," "I really care about these animals," and "I have gotten through a lot, and I can get through this." These are just ideas. Some people excel with words, while others excel with pictures. Have some fun here while you create this grounding mechanism.

2. Write, draw, or tape this to an index card. If it is memory or a hug or something less tangible, write out a reminder of it.

3. Breathe in for a quick count of 2 and then breathe out for a long exhale.

4. Pull up your pictures or words for a quick moment.

5. Look at the animal and the decision, and check your knowledge that we did earlier.

6. Notice if you feel different about the current case.

7. Trust yourself. (This is the hardest step and takes tons of practice.)

REFERENCE

Dickson, B. (2023). Ethical dilemmas and moral distress in companion animal veterinary medicine: Mental health implications. Unpublished manuscript. Chrome-extension://efaidnbmnnnibpcajpcglcle findmkaj/https://scholars.wlu.ca/cgi/viewcontent. cgi?article=3771&context=etd

CHAPTER 21

Sleep

Sleep is important. It makes our brains and bodies work better. You can argue that there is no time for sleep, you have to get one more thing done, or you can't sleep anyway, so there is no point. Making sleep a priority can make all the other things work much better. It can feel like staying up late to get work done is worth it. It will reduce stress in the morning if you get things done. However, the reality is that lack of sleep actually creates more stress in your day. Chemicals released in the body in response to sleep deprivation mimic those of stress responses, meaning that staying awake can actually create more stress (Lo Martire *et al.*, 2024). Look back on the days you stayed awake to get caught up. Did you feel better the next day? There is always something to do. Did you feel like you caught up on your work? In the long term, did it work?

It is also true that when we are stressed, we do not sleep as well (Zhang *et al.*, 2024). It can be easy to justify that you would struggle either way. The solution would be to manage your stress throughout the day, so that you can sleep more effectively at night and, therefore, manage your stress more effectively the next day. It is all a difficult cycle, I know. The need to sleep is not isolated to humans. Animals need sleep, too. In horses and dogs, sleep significantly impacts their ability to learn new skills, remember patterns taught to them, and work at a steady pace. Why do we feel like we are different? (Barbosa *et al.*, 2024).

Sometimes we argue that we cannot sleep because we finally have time to relax, and we need to savor it. It feels nice to veg out and relax. However, it takes a toll on your body. It becomes harder to relax throughout the day due to the stress hormones that come with being tired, and then you feel like you need it more at night. It becomes another vicious cycle.

REWRITING SLEEP SCHEDULE

Deciding that sleep is a priority and you would like to get more sleep can be a difficult process. If you are accustomed to avoiding sleep in some way, it can be challenging to teach your body that sleep is actually essential. As people prioritize sleep, they may become anxious about getting and staying asleep. Their body may also be used to not sleeping at a greater level. There are several ways to create better sleep patterns, but all require some effort and may be uncomfortable. One Idea is to reset your sleep schedule using cognitive behavioral therapy (CBT) for insomnia (Spielman and Bottin, 1993). This sleep routine has been used for people moving from night shifts to day shifts, adjusting to time zones, and finding a sleep schedule. This method can be very difficult because you will likely be very tired throughout the process. This is a high-level breakdown of the concept.

EXERCISE 21.1 Setting a healthy sleep schedule

1. Decide what you would like your sleep schedule to look like. Consider what a healthy amount of sleep is, what is realistic with your schedule, and something you can maintain consistency with.

2. Notice how long you typically sleep a night. If you usually sleep for 5 hours from 12 to 5, we will start with this.

3. Only lie in bed for the 5 hours allotted.

4. If you wake up and cannot go back to sleep, be sure to leave the bed and return to try again.

5. As you can lie in bed for the whole time, increase this by 15–20 minutes until you get to a place where you are comfortable and rested.

6. Once you feel rested throughout the day and comfortable with your sleep schedule, it is important to adhere to it as closely as possible. If you get off, you will likely revert to your old patterns and have to go through this process again. It is a lot of work, making it more motivating to stay on your schedule (even on days you are not working).

SLEEP HYGIENE

Sleep hygiene is extremely important in creating healthy sleeping patterns. It can be tempting to doom scroll yourself to sleep (which doesn't really work), fall asleep on the couch watching TV, or fly by the seat of your pants when deciding when to sleep. If this approach is not working for you and you struggle to sleep, I encourage you to try applying sleep hygiene techniques to see if it makes a difference. Here are some key points to keep in mind when trying to get enough sleep. These things can help you fall and stay asleep more effectively.

- Avoid substances that are not prescribed. You may think you sleep better when you are drinking alcohol, but it is a less restful sleep, and it gets in the way of sleep in the long term.

- Avoid screens at night. The blue light emitted by screens can trick your brain into thinking the sun is still out, producing serotonin (the neurotransmitter that keeps you awake) and depleting melatonin (the neurotransmitter that helps you fall asleep), ultimately disrupting sleep cycles. Consider relaxing with an audiobook, a guided meditation, or a paper book to read.

- If you are anxious about falling asleep, it will be more difficult to do so. Allow yourself time in bed to relax your body without trying to fall asleep. You can do this with your favorite breathing exercise, a guided meditation, or a visualization. If you become stressed about falling asleep, stop trying to fall asleep and start working on relaxing your body during that time. You may trick your body into falling asleep, but it also creates space for the sleeplessness to be productive.

- Have a bedtime routine. Make sure this is something you do every night as a ritual to signal to your body that it's time for bed. Maybe you shut down the house, brush your teeth, wash your face, fluff your pillow, and then lie down. It does not matter what the routine is or how long it takes, but it is helpful to have some routine that tells your body that it is time to sleep.

- If you wake up in the middle of the night and cannot go to sleep, give yourself 15 more minutes. This does not have to be exact, as it is not helpful to look at your phone, but rather a basic idea. If you are still not asleep, get up and do something small. Get a drink of water, go to the bathroom, just something that allows your body to reset, and try to sleep again. Give yourself 30 more minutes of relaxing in bed (not worrying about sleeping, just spending time relaxing). If you are still not asleep, get up and do something. Wipe a countertop, rearrange something small, or step outside. Find something that doesn't require too much attention, doesn't involve a screen, and is pretty boring. Lie back down with the intention of relaxing.

- If you are a visual person, this exercise may be helpful in promoting sleep. Visualize a chalkboard or whiteboard. Write a word, any word, on the board visually. It could be the word that is bothering you, or the word sleep, or just your name. Try writing the word as slowly as you can. Once you have written the word, erase it and write your next word, as slowly as you can. This makes the eyes move as if they are sleeping in REM cycle and also creates a distraction from worry thoughts if you concentrate on it hard enough.

- Your brain is filled with a million thoughts about your day, what you should do tomorrow, and other worries that get in the way of sleep. Our brain can actually only think about one thing at a time. Give yourself space to think of something relaxing. Some people visualize their thoughts floating away on clouds or a leaf on the river. Some fill their brain with counting their breath (1 for a breath in, 2 for a breath out), while others will simply count 1 and 2 and start over. Some give themselves a different number. Counting sheep is a thing because it fills your brain with something else to think about.

- Try not to be frantic about falling asleep. Sometimes we become so anxious about needing sleep and not wanting to waste our time in bed that we wind ourselves up trying to fall asleep. Allowing yourself space to sleep as much as you can during the time you set aside for sleep and accepting that sleep may be difficult as you reestablish the habit is very important.

- Ensure your bed is reserved only for sleep. If you lie in bed and watch TV, scrolling your phone, or reading books, the bed becomes a space for this instead of sleep, meaning your body does not relax when it lies in bed. When the bed is only used for sleep, your body associates it with relaxing.

EXERCISE 21.2   Progressive body relaxation

This technique is a great way to distract yourself from thoughts and spend time relaxing your body, rather than falling asleep. I provide examples on how to tighten each group for those who might not know how, but if you have a different method for tightening a muscle group, I encourage you to try it. As you go through each section of your body, you will pull on an inhale and release on an exhale. You can do this once or multiple times. If you have an injury or pain, skip that part.

1. Start with your toes. As you breathe in, tighten your toes by curling them; as you exhale, release them.

2. Move up to your calves. Tighten your calves by pulling your toes up. On an exhale, release them.

3. Now move on to each muscle group through out your whole body.

   a. Your upper legs (pulling up on them)
   b. your glutes (squeeze your cheeks together)
   c. your abdominal muscles(suck in and pull your stomach up toward your ribs)
   d. Your chest (Bring your shoulders in, then again bring your shoulders back).
   e. upper arms(pull your arms up as if you are showing off your biceps)
   f. lower arms (Pull your hand in toward the inner part of your elbow)
   g. Hands (clench them as tight as you can)
   h. Shoulders (Shrug)
   i. Face (Squish your face as much as you can)

4. Now tighten all the muscles in your body that you can on the inhale and release them on the exhale.

REFERENCES

Barbosa, Â. P. *et al.* (2024). 'Sleep pattern interference in the cognitive performance of Lusitano horses', *Animals*, 14(2), p. 334.

Lo Martire, V., Berteotti, C., Zoccoli, G. and Bastianini, S. (2024). 'Improving sleep to improve stress resilience', *Current Sleep Medicine Reports*, 10(1), pp. 23–33.

Spielman, A. J. and Bottin, D. (1993). 'Cognitive-behavior therapy for late-life insomnia', *Sleep*, 16(5), pp. 491–496.

Zhang, J. *et al.* (2024). 'Effects of stress on sleep quality: Multiple mediating effects of rumination and social anxiety', *Psicologia: Reflexão e Crítica*, 37(1), p. 10.

Making It Through Difficult Times

CHAPTER 22

MAKING IT THROUGH A MISTAKE

Yews phew, is this a difficult one? When a big mistake is made, the emotions can be extreme. It can be difficult to use any skill at all. I know that we are always saying "everyone makes mistakes, be easy on yourself," but when a big mistake is made, and there are consequences to this mistake, boy, can it be overwhelming. It is easy to fear your job, your career, your sense of self, or all the things. Many people become disconnected, questioning their purpose, abilities, and career. Being realistic about this can be essential in surviving it. The last thing you need is to feel terrible about your mistake, while also feeling shame for feeling terrible, because you are supposed to forgive yourself. Mistakes are difficult in any field. Medical fields carry an additional burden due to a genuine fear of losing their job over a grievance, as well as concern for those being treated. The thing is, a mistake (even a large one) does not mean you are bad at what you do; it means you made a mistake. Because you care about the animals you treat, most veterinarians (especially young ones) have a great fear that they will be ineffective in their work. A mistake can reinforce this belief. So, as many times as I remind you that mistakes are a natural part of being human, you may not believe me.

Thought questioning can be helpful in these situations, although it can also be terribly difficult. If you can think of specific events that contradict the belief that is arising for you (e.g., "I am stupid," "I am worthless," and "I am a bad person"), that is great. Specific events may be moments when you felt smart, especially accomplished, or proud of yourself. For instance, if the brief is that you are a bad surgeon, you would think about all the times when you were really a great surgeon, and things went really well for you.

Thought questioning is an incredible skill, but when the emotion is that large, it gets more complicated. A first step in the process is to recognize that you are grieving. This grief can get pretty complicated because it is unclear exactly what you are grieving. When the thing you are grieving is less clear, it can also feel weird to call it grief. A step would be to explore whether you are grieving and what you are grieving about. Sometimes people grieve the loss of a belief. If you thought it could never happen to you, you may grieve that this can no longer be a belief. If you reached out for support and did not receive it, you may grieve that the system did not meet your expectations or hopes. If the mistake is egregious enough, you may grieve the fact that a formal complaint may be placed against you. If the mistake was made because of a lack of resources, you may grieve that the resources are not available. The grieving brain, by Mary Frances O'Connor (2022), explains grief as a difficulty for the brain to understand that something has changed. When a person dies, our brain is adjusting to them not being there anymore. This also means that our brain has the potential to react in the same way to any significant change. Give yourself time with your grief.

Find the people who are willing to support you fully. When we go through difficult times, especially ones that bring up shame and grief, it is very tempting to isolate. However, isolation actually exacerbates these moments. If your employer is being hard on you, it may be important to take a break from your employer (family medical leave may be necessary if your reaction is very large). If your colleagues are telling you that you should be kinder to yourself, and it is excruciatingly difficult, let them know this is not helpful. Take a moment, slow down, and ask yourself, "What do I need right now?" Ask this question several times. Your first instinct responses may not be very kind, but if you get past these initial responses, you may find that you have an answer to whether you need alone time or to be surrounded by others.

You may not even know what support looks like. A fundamental answer is that you need time. Allow time to be sad, mad, or whatever emotion you need regarding the incident. Also know that even though it feels like the pain is inevitable for the rest of your life, you can make it through this difficult time if you give yourself time and space. Emotional wounds need time in the same way physical wounds need time to heal; we just forget that they are similar.

During moments of crisis, such as those that can arise from making a mistake, your amygdala goes into hyperdrive, trying to protect you from anything that could harm you. It is essential to acknowledge that when the amygdala is highly activated, it shuts down the decision-making part of the brain, making it challenging, if not impossible, to perceive all aspects of the event, oneself, and day-to-day life. Knowing that you may not be able to see all of the facts right now can be helpful in allowing you to give yourself time to see what is actually true instead of what feels true.

When managing the aftereffects of a big mistake, it can be easy to forget your purpose. It is also important to define the purpose you have on this planet. If you did not go into veterinary medicine, who would miss out? If your response is "no one, they would be better off without me," that is your amygdala speaking. There are many animals that may not have received quality care if you had never become a veterinarian. Keep asking the question until you can answer from a place of reflection instead of destruction. Eventually, as you heal, I hope that you can recognize the amazing impact you make on this world in whatever way, shape, form, or fashion that may be for you.

Outside of working through your own difficult reaction to a mistake, it is important to check if a repair is needed. Do you need to apologize to anyone? This apology can be conveyed through a letter (whether sent or not), a gift, or a conversation. If a repair needs to be made, it can be very healing to initiate the repair process. This can also be very scary because just because you make the effort for a repair, it does not mean the receiver has to accept it. Find a way to initiate repair that is safe for you. If you cannot make contact with the person (or animal) you need to repair with, or if it is just too scary, it is okay to write a letter that is never sent. There is something important about going through the motions of repair, even if it is not done in person. It is also important to repair with yourself. Consider writing a letter to yourself, forgiving yourself for the mistake you made and reminding yourself of the lessons you learned. Maybe acknowledge the grief and give it a name. Maybe you just free-flow write and see what comes up.

Eventually, it is important to reach a point where you can learn from your mistakes. Look at what led to the mistake and determine if you can shield yourself from this in the future. Were you overworked and tired? Were you asked to perform a procedure that you were less familiar with without supervision? Were you burnt-out, stressed, or overwhelmed, causing your frontal cortex to work less effectively? Give yourself space to remember that all of these things can play a role in mistakes. This gives you space to remember that this space happened for a reason. It can help you become a better person in the future.

SUMMARY ABOUT SURVIVING A LARGE MISTAKE

These steps do not have to be done in order. Large emotions are a personal process, and I encourage you to do them in the order that works best for you.

Step 1: Grieve. This is a sad event. Allow yourself some space to grieve. The key here is to allow it to come in bursts instead of tsunamis. You can do this by setting aside scheduled grief time, and when the grief comes up, remind yourself to save it for grief time. If you choose this way, make sure the grief time is contained (for example: I will grieve at 7:00 a.m. and again at 3:00 p.m. and if you need to add one more at 6:00 p.m. I will grieve for 40 minutes and fully think about how sad this is. When the 40-minute timer goes off, I will find some way to fully distract from it. Another way to do this would be to set aside distraction time. When I feel overwhelmed by grief, I will play Tetris on my phone and then get up and take a shower or wash my face. I will go back to the grief after I give it a moment. You can play with what makes sense to you, given your grief process.

Step 2: Check to see if a repair is needed. Do you need to apologize to anyone? This apology can be done through a letter (you send or do not send), a gift, or a conversation. If a repair needs to be made, it can be very healing to start the process of repair. Find a way to initiate repair that is safe for you. If you cannot make contact with the person (or animal) you need to repair with, or if it is just too scary, it is okay to write a letter that is never sent. There is something important about going through the motions of repair, even if it is not done in person.

Step 3: Repair with yourself. Find a way to learn something new. This allows you to be more than the mistake. You still have a brain, and you can still do better. Your something new can be related to the mistake, or it can be unrelated.

Step 4: Talk to people who are safe to talk to about this. Colleagues, mentors, or a therapist are a great place to start. As the great Brene Brown's research states, the best antidote to shame is being vulnerable with people who will be in your court (Brown, 2015).

Step 5: Take your time. You do not have to rush the process of forgiving yourself. It can be a painful process with no defined timeframe. If the process makes you want to leave the field or make large decisions in your life, take your time with that as well. Remember that when we talk about well-being, slow is fast. This can be hard to hear when you are in pain, but it is extremely important. Rushing the process tells your body it is unsafe, and this leads to even longer processing and many times more intense emotions. If your only option feels like taking your life, please find the support you need. Give yourself a chance to heal before you give up.

MAKING IT THROUGH A FRANTIC DAY

Frantic days happen, no matter how grounded you are or how many skills you are using; there is always a day, or many, when the scheduling is beyond full. There are days when a simple case is more complicated than you ever thought. The animal whose temperament does not match their lab work, and you feel stuck. The day when one or many people call in sick, and you are short-staffed. You are running around with your hair on fire. Everyone seems to be on edge on days like these. I have never met anyone who is not impacted by a frantic day at all. Instead of being hard on yourself that skills fell short and you lost your temper (or whatever your go-to response is for stress), pause and recognize that days happen. Your nervous system is naturally on fire when the world is on fire around you. Slowing down becomes unsafe. We can logically say this is not true and that if you slowed down, you would make fewer mistakes, be kinder to colleagues and handlers, and leave the day feeling much better. However, logic is not always the deciding factor here, and sometimes our body system just doesn't listen. This is where acceptance plays a crucial role more than anything else. However, there are still micro-skills that you can use to keep you from being over the edge and frantic. The key is to practice these skills on days that are a little faster-paced, so that they can be effective on days that are full-on frantic. Practicing tells your nervous system that these work, so that you are more likely to use them by accident on the frantic days when you really need them. Below are a few breathing techniques you can use during a frantic day to nurture your nervous system on the move. I like breathing techniques these days because you have to breathe anyway, you might as well make it productive. You don't have to stop moving for these, making it more likely that you will actually do them.

EXERCISE 22.1 Pause in your breath

---

1. Take a moment and notice how you are breathing naturally. Just right now, as you read this book

2. Notice how deep or shallow your natural breath is. Notice how quick or slow it is.

3. Give your breath just a moment to settle in.

4. Now notice the natural pause at the top and bottom of your breath. Everyone has it. Continue to breathe normally, bringing your attention to the pause.

   Now you know that the pause exists, it's time to use it as a micro skill.

5. Pauses happen when you do not even realize they are there. You have natural pauses each time you change tasks in the same way that you have pauses in your breath. Start noticing these tiny pauses in your day. All you have to do is notice them. If you want to make a game out of it, see if you can count how many pauses you have in a day (there are a lot you probably will struggle to get an actual number—it's just a game). These pauses are very small, but just like there needs to be a pause to transition from inhaling to exhaling, there also needs to be a pause to move from one case to the next.

As you start to notice pauses in your day, you will also begin to see them on frantic days, which tells your body that you are transitioning, naturally slowing down your responses so that you can be more effective, no matter how wild the world around you seems to be.

EXERCISE 22.2 Finding the exhale

Throughout the day, your body constantly activates and relaxes through your breath. When you exhale, you relax. When you inhale, you activate. You need both- or you have some real problems. When life gets busy, we are prone to holding our breath or inhaling more as our body believes we need to be more activated. This is why people sigh when they are annoyed or stressed. It is the body's way of saying it is exhausted from inhaling too much and needs a big exhale.

1. Before you leave for the day, as you leave the door of the clinic or while you get in your car, let out a huge intentional sigh.

2. Notice what happens.

3. Find a cue to begin exhaling more regularly throughout the day.

Along the same idea, some people yawn more when emotions are more intense or when they are stressed. This is the body's way of activating even more, as it is a large inhale. It is also why we yawn when we are tired, if you are starting to feel shut down during these days.

1. Force yourself to yawn.

2. Just notice

3. If you are noticing a lot of yawns naturally, notice the need to inhale.

EXERCISE 22.3   Evening your breath

Knowing that your breathing is likely not in an even pattern when you are stressed is important. Practice this breathing as you walk between clinic rooms on a busy day.

1. Create an even cadence for your breathing. In a perfectly regulated world, this would be five counts in and five counts out. However, this may be anxiety-provoking to some people. For this reason, I think it is important to give yourself flexibility. Allow yourself to decide what feels best for your body. I do not recommend less than a three-count as this could foster more panic, as it looks a lot like hyperventilating. I also do not recommend more than 5, as this may relax you too much, and you do need some activation to make it through the day.

2. Continue to breathe in for a count of five and out for a count of five (or whatever cadence you decided) for six sets of breaths.

3. You do not have to slow your thoughts or your body for this. You are only concentrating on your breath.

4. Notice if there is any change to your nervous system.

   As you try out these skills, be mindful of the fact that each one of them is designed to reduce franticness; however, your body needs some level of franticness when the day is genuinely chaotic. Because of this, it likely will not allow you to relax all the way, nor do you want it to. You just need it to stay within its window. This way, you are less likely to make mistakes or produce unnecessary long-term stress. (Edwards, 2016).

EXERCISE 22.4   Square breathing

Some people benefit more from a square breathing technique. This technique allows space to reset breath patterns when the cadenced breathing is too difficult.

1. Breathe in for a count of four

2. Hold your breath for a count of four

3. Breathe out for a count of four

4. Hold your breath for a count of four

5. Repeat this four times (or however many you are willing to before you get distracted from the chaos of the day.

EXERCISE 22.5   The reset breath

Have you ever noticed that when a young child is throwing a tantrum, they will sometimes take a deep breath in during the fit, and then calm down for a bit? It is the body's way of resetting and activating itself during extreme emotions. We can trick our bodies and reset similarly.

1. Take two large, quick inhales.

2. Exhale as slowly and as long as you can

3. Notice if you feel a difference

SURVIVING A TOXIC WORK ENVIRONMENT

Regardless of your field, it is likely that you have had, will have, or currently have a toxic supervisor. Sometimes this is due to toxic management styles. I have noticed a movement of management styles that can be compared to bullying, more managers picking on people because of personality differences vs. performance issues. I am not saying this is across the board; I am simply saying I notice it with people who come into my office in distress. I am not sure these supervisors know how people internalize this mistreatment. When you bully someone and set them up for failure, the effects can linger into personal life and the next job. Feelings of not being good enough are common when leaving an environment like this. People are wondering if that person was correct or if it is their fault that the job failed. While management style can sometimes be toxic, at other times, the toxicity is not anyone's fault. As humans, we like to blame people. It feels like someone should be at fault. Sometimes, the manager does not want to acknowledge their own flaws, so they place them on others. While this is not their fault, I sure wish they would get help for it. Sometimes the management style reminds us of someone from the past who was toxic in our lives. We may not notice a connection, but we struggle to be in the same room as them, as they trigger past memories and reactions. Sometimes the management style just doesn't jive, and for some reason, it hits us in a funny way. It honestly doesn't matter whose fault it is or why the environment is toxic for us. Sometimes toxicity does not come from management; it comes from colleagues. These colleagues may be responding to their own work-related stress. They may have their own story that makes them difficult to work with, or they may remind you of someone you have not liked in the past. If you find yourself in a situation where a workplace triggers you, and you notice reactions to your work and the people you work with, I encourage you to take a few steps to see if this is a situation you should leave or stay in.

EXERCISE 22.6	Deciding if you should stay or leave

1. Remind yourself that everyone is doing the best that they can. This does not mean that they cannot do better; in fact, you, me, and everyone else can do better. We are all doing the best we can with what we have today, and hopefully, we will learn more to do better. Your boss and all your co-workers are doing the best they can.

2. Utilize the skills that speak to you most to ground yourself. Doing this exercise in a state of resentment or out of your window does not work as well.

3. Check in on this person's point of view, without your own perspective in it. What are the supervisor's primary values? What do they fear? Make some assumptions about them based on what you know so that you can put yourself in their shoes. Do the same if a colleague is the culprit for toxicity.

4. Practice communicating with the person using their language in whatever way you can, without giving up your own purpose and values. See what it looks like to ask for your needs in a different way.

5. Check in with yourself. When you are working, are you working from your own values and morals? When you fact-check, are you doing a good job? Where are you exceeding and where are you thriving from your own perspective, not anyone else's? If you made positive changes toward improvement, would it be accepted in this environment?

6. Are things improving with these altered viewpoints? If not, it may be time to consider moving on and finding a new job. This can be terrifying, coming from a toxic supervisor situation. There is a feeling that this is "the devil that you know." What if you leave and it is the same or worse? What if they are right and you can't cut it? I encourage you to explore options and try them out. In my experience, most people leave and find a much better fit when the situation is truly toxic.

FAQ ABOUT LEAVING A WORK ENVIRONMENT

1. **What if I leave and jump into another toxic relationship with my superiors?**

   I cannot promise that you won't, but I can say it is not as likely. Because of your experience in this toxic environment, you learned a specific personality type that you are less likely to get along with. When you interview, it is more likely you will recognize this personality before it happens again. Sometimes the environment changed: it was the perfect fit before, but it's not now, and you may have a difficult time trusting the goodness of the next job. Remind yourself that you can enjoy the good, and you will notice the toxic much sooner now. Make a list of questions that are important to you as you interview. Maybe how they manage difficult personalities in a clinic? What are the primary values affecting your role? Maybe what does support look like? Compare what you do not want in your next job to your current situation and ask questions based on this information.

2. **What if this pays way better than a situation that might be better?**

   I call this the gold handcuffs. You cannot leave a position because of the pay. I encourage you to ask yourself if you can truly afford a pay cut to be happier. If the answer is no, it is important to label the environment as toxic in your head, arm yourself with an arsenal of all the skills you have, knowing you are going to need them, and constantly remind yourself "What is mine and what is theirs?" Label their why in your head, even though you disagree with it, to remind yourself they are doing the best they can, even if you wish they were doing better. You may even need a mantra to remind yourself that you are dealing with this crappy situation for the money. At one point in my career, I was unable to leave my position that was not a good fit because I needed the money. I would sing "Money Money Money" by ABBA in my head to humorify it and remind myself of my why. Don't forget your values that apply to the field, and search for things that align with your values and give you energy. Notice the parts of the job that you enjoy and feel good at. When you find them, try to notice them mentally. If you have the power, make sure to throw those moments in after predictably difficult ones, such as meetings with the toxic person.

3. **What if I am actually kinda mediocre or worse, bad, at my job?**

   I am going to be honest, I do not know you, and so I cannot tell you that you are good at your job; that would be misleading at best. What I can tell you is that you are probably good at some part of your job and could use improvement in others. Look at the places where you are doing well and take note of them. They are hard to notice when things get hard. Even if there is a "but" in the way, give yourself space to notice them anyway. Look at the places you can improve. Decide if that is a growth area you are interested in gaining more knowledge about, or if it is something to accept. If you need to gain more knowledge, I hope that you do that. If you decide to accept it, find ways to work around it by utilizing your strengths. Are the complaints of the toxic person valid when you truly check the facts from a very logical standpoint? If the answer is yes, explore ways to grow and improve. If the answer is no, this may be a moment where it is about them more than you. Trust that even though it doesn't feel true and it can be scary to believe, maybe you are doing just fine or even really good.

4. **Is human medicine better?**

   When people start to notice work-related stressors and toxic environments, they often want to run away. Remember, the job becomes a sabretooth tiger, and I can tell you right now, if a sabretooth tiger walked into this room right now, I would be running. I hear this a lot from struggling veterinary professionals. This concept involves leaving the field or pursuing a career in human medicine. Many even do. If you are making this decision based on work-related stress or a potentially toxic work environment, I encourage you to work through the yuck before making the decision. You may still decide to leave, but you've worked really hard to get here, and I encourage you to give it a full shot first.

5. **People around me don't seem to get it? They keep telling me to get over it and leave. How can I communicate in a way that allows me to get support from others?**

   When work is toxic, it is common to complain about it regularly. I have done it, people around me have done it, clients have done it, and most people do. Unfortunately, it is likely the same complaint over and over again, which can be very exhausting for those around us. People can get exhausted and simply tell you to stay or leave, but pick one, which can feel invalidating. When discussing your situation with others, it can be helpful to journal first or sit with the situation while practicing grounding exercises. This allows you to decide what you want from the conversation, making it more productive for the person you are talking to. You can decide, do I just need to vent, do I need affirmation that it is as crazy as I think it is, and do I need permission to do something, or act in a certain way? Knowing your intention can direct the conversation in a way that is less frustrating to both you and the person you are talking to. If the answer is that you just need to vent, let the person know this, so that they know their role is not to problem solve, and they can feel less frustrated with the situation. The first couple of times you do this, you may get the need wrong and only realize when the person gives you what you asked for that this was not actually what you were looking for. That is okay, you will get better at it, just keep practicing.

6. How do I know if I should stick it out and keep trying these steps, and when I should call it quits and start looking?

    That is the question that often haunts people when they are coming from toxicity. When is it finally time to stop trying? The answer is honestly up to you. Give yourself some steps or a time limit that is reasonable. During that time limit (Maybe a month or two) try not to ask if you will leave. Simply ask if you can use the skills. Mark the date on your calendar. When it comes up, take some time to review your last few months. Journal about all the ways you have made changes and how the job has responded. If it has not improved, it's time to leave, no matter how scary it might be. Giving yourself these rigid guidelines can be very helpful because it takes the emotion out of the decision-making and gives you a reason to make a decision. Often, the most challenging part of decision-making is the wavering; the follow-through is often much easier.

7. What if they fire me?

    Being fired can add a whole new layer of difficulty to the challenges that arise from a toxic work environment. Nasty self-talk can really kick in when we find ourselves in these situations. Please ensure you find people who can support you during this time and affirm you if needed. If you genuinely believe that you deserved to be fired and were not being your best self, learn from that experience and decide what you need to improve on in your next job. If you know in some part of you that this was unjust, please write this down. The truth can get really covered up by negative self-talk in these situations. Having it written in your handwriting allows for a valid argument when the negative thoughts get worse. Structure and plan your day, you are used to a very fast-paced, structured environment. Write out your schedule for job searching, self-growth, and relaxation so that it is harder to fall into depression with natural self-talk that comes with it.

8. What if I can't find a job?

    Job searching can be excruciatingly difficult. It is filled with rejection and sometimes unknowns. I encourage you to keep trying, no matter how hard it is, but remember that it can be difficult due to rejection. Give yourself space to do things you are good at during this time. This can counteract the rejection. If you are still working, it can feel like you don't have time for this, but creating even moments for things you are good at is essential in these moments. If you are depressed, you may not find enjoyment in the task, but do it anyway. It creates some space to fight the crummy feelings that come with rejection. In the meantime, equip yourself with an arsenal of skills, establish a schedule for applying them, and be aware that it will be challenging for the duration of your search. Developing skills and acknowledging the difficult is exhausting, but living in a toxic work environment with nothing to show for it is even more exhausting.

LINGERING EFFECTS OF A TOXIC WORK ENVIRONMENT

Let's say you do all the work, decide it is time to leave, gain the courage, find another job, and leave. Sometimes, just moving to a safe environment and starting over is all you need. Sometimes those nasty, negative thoughts come in, and just don't seem to leave. You find yourself having a hard time trusting the goodness of the next place. You wonder about your place in a healthy work environment. You question your strengths and abilities based on your past employer. Some people even have complete trauma responses with nightmares, ruminating thoughts, reliving the past workplace, avoiding things that remind them of the past workplace, and constant fear. What do you do when you find yourself having a difficult time figuring out how to settle in a non-toxic work environment? There are two ways to address this issue. I would recommend having a therapist in your back pocket in a situation like this. Sometimes we can work this through on our own using information from this book and what we have learned in other places. Sometimes it is deeper, and our body system just can't find safety without a third party helping.

Have you ever noticed that the most significant changes happen within crisis situations? Change can happen outside of a crisis as well, which is much more comfortable, but a crisis seems to bring change. It took such extreme discomfort at your last job that you made the change to move to this job. This can be a great opportunity to create routines that build your well-being and resilience. When you move jobs, there is a settling period anyway. You have a new set of routines, meet new people, learn new systems, and, at the very least, drive to a new place. Why not add in some new routine while you are at it? This can be finding your cue to check in with yourself as you get used to your new environment. Developing a grounding routine during your commute home can create space for resilience. Use this time to ground and establish how you would like to be at the new job. Concentrating on you and the things that you can do allows space for your body to recognize that, in this situation, you have control over your safety. You start to let your body know that you are indeed safe and have escaped the toxic environment.

You may also need to focus intensely on your thoughts to get through this challenging time. It can be hard because our thoughts can be so strong that they feel true. You have to work really hard to alter your thoughts in a way that you can use the new position as a way to restart. Your body and mind may fight you extremely hard to get you to a place where you can navigate this process. Here are some steps they can help with the thoughts themselves.

EXERCISE 22.7 For making it through the lingering effects of a past job

1. Notice that you are stuck in a pattern of negative self-talk and are emotionally vulnerable. If you are not aware of your patterns, they can be difficult to address. Acknowledging that you are going through a hard time also communicates to us that we need to use more skills.

2. Call the thoughts what they are. "This is from the past job, I do not know if it is true right now," is an example of a way that you can label these thoughts and reactions. Notice that I am not encouraging full-on arguing with it. Because our thoughts come from the safety response I spoke about before, if we fully argue with them, they can dig in their heels and get bigger as if to say, "Hey, if you don't listen to me, you might die." Plus, we cannot tell the future, so if you say, "This is a completely safe place where nothing bad can happen," your body system knows you cannot tell the future and ramps up its reactions because you are not listening.

3. Start checking the facts. Are you really as bad as you think you are? What are you good at right now? Is this the last work environment where it is hard to trust the good? How can you challenge these thoughts with facts? Point out ways in

which this supervisor is different than the last. Notice if the people you work with respond differently to you and the situations they are working in. Become focused on what is different, so that your body knows you are in a different environment and can adapt accordingly.

4. Remind your body that you are now in a safer environment and list out the things that make the environment safe. Remember, your body will argue with you if you don't provide it with facts. Make sure these facts are actual and based on the observations you made in step 3.

Even with skills, a therapist, and all the tools in the toolbox of well-being, it can still take time to adjust to a new environment adequately. It may take months to reach a point where you truly trust that the new environment does not harbor the same toxicity as the old one. I encourage you to acknowledge that this is a hard season and that with really quality skills, you can make it through this and enjoy your job again. It is possible. The field of veterinary medicine is becoming less and less toxic. This is a huge relief. But that does not mean that toxicity does not exist. It exists in all fields. You do not have to endure a toxic work environment; there are many safe environments available to you.

THE DREADED ONLINE REVIEW

When I am talking to veterinary professionals, online reviews are the number one thing that gets in the way of setting boundaries. Human doctors have less of a fear of the online reviews, and I am not sure why. There are trolls on the internet. There are people on this planet who are entitled. The internet makes these people's opinions heard more than ever before. It can be heartbreaking to work extremely hard for a pet only to log on to your favorite platform and see that the owner has complained about you in a public forum. What is even scarier to some is the format that is public, but which you don't see. Social media posts about the bad experience that you cannot see.

You have enough pressure in this field to let this bother you, but it still does. Most people reading reviews are actually going to read reviews, not just look at stars. If there are 10 great or mostly good reviews and one bad review that appears to be from someone who is just angry, they will focus on the great reviews. If they do not, you may not want them as a customer. If someone is yelling and screaming at you, and you ask them to leave, and they send you a bad review. Let them. I know this is easier said than done, but it is very important that you know that reviews are often not a reflection of you and your business. If you are getting many bad reviews and a few good reviews, it might be time to look at your customer service. If you receive many positive reviews and a few negative ones, focus on the people who are praising you and want you to succeed. It might even be helpful not to check the reviews at all. If you grow your business based on care for the animals and their handlers and treat people with respect, while asking others to treat you with respect as well, you can leave your day feeling like you are really successful in your business.

It might be hard to hear this advice. I am basically just saying F*ck 'em and move on. Easier said than done, I know. Veterinary professionals like to do things correctly, and a negative review might as well be a C on a paper. It feels like the worst thing that could happen. However, you do not have control over other people. Acknowledging that you have control over yourself and your practices can be very helpful in letting the other stuff go. It is also important to acknowledge that you are just as important as your clients when we consider this in a broader context. We are all humans, we all have loved ones, we all do important things, and when all is said and done, no one is truly more important than anyone else. (Value and belief of mine, you don't have to hold it.) It can often be easier to see customers as more important than you are (Maybe because of the stinking internet), but please remember that you are just as important. You deserve to be treated with respect, you deserve to charge what you need to keep your business successful, and you deserve to have a professional opinion about the animals you serve. If people don't like that, they can send the review and move on.

Being firm in your values and mission as a veterinarian can be very helpful in this regard. If you have a strong basis for why you perform in the way that you do as a clinic and as a person, you are more likely to perform with consistency and confidence that you are making a decision based on what is important, not a review (unless your primary goal is to have only positive reviews—that's a tough one).

EXERCISE 22.8 Surviving a negative review

1. Take a deep, calming breath and exhale slowly before reading the review. Good or Bad. We want to make sure we are not starting in a place of emotion; they have the potential to be big enough as we read.

2. Read the review.

3. Take another breath. If it is one that activates you a ton, set it down and take a quick stroll, push on a wall, or do whatever skill you like to do best.

4. Fact-check the review. Is there anything that you can do better? Is there any validity to what they are saying? Would changes benefit the clinic as a whole or just this person? If there is any validity to the review, create a list of steps to implement the change; if not, there is not much to do in this step.

5. Go through and read some of the positive reviews that you have gotten in the past. Remind yourself that it is not just this angry person who rules the internet.

6. Determine whether it is effective to respond if it is a forum that requires a response. If you do decide to respond, please make sure you are validating and offering a solution to their problem. It is also okay just to let it be and not respond. I have seen both sides of this argument.

7. If it does not require any action, take a breath and be grateful that this person will no longer be visiting your clinic and treating you and your staff with disrespect.

8. Move forward, providing the best care possible for the animals and handlers that come into your clinic.

Sometimes the clinic is more worried about reviews than you are. This can lead to a company policy that makes it difficult to establish clear boundaries and serve the animals and their handlers in the best possible way. It can be helpful to discuss these concepts with the people who hold power, provided they are willing to listen. Either way, you can still use the skills discussed in this chapter. Allow yourself the space to notice the successes and strengths you have in the workplace and check the validity of the complaints and reviews. Make changes where they need to be made, while trying to remember that making a change does not mean you did a bad job; it simply means you are continuing to grow.

REFERENCES

Brown, B. (2015). *Daring greatly: How the courage to be vulnerable transforms the way we live, love, parent, and lead.* New York: Avery, an imprint of Penguin Random House.

Edwards, S. D. (2016). 'Influence of HeartMath quick coherence technique on psychophysiological coherence and feeling states', *African Journal for Physical Activity and Health Sciences*, 22(4:1), pp. 1006–1018.

O'Connor, M.-F. (2022). *The grieving brain.* Hollywood, CA: O'Connor Production Inc.

Conclusion

As you digest all of the information from the book you may feel overwhelmed about how the future will look. Maybe you fear it will be temporary and you will not be able to apply it long term. Maybe it was difficult to actually carry out the skills and you are worried you will never be able to make change. Maybe you are a student or a young professional and you are terrified about what the future brings. However you are sitting with the material please know that change can happen and you can succeed. This section of the book will review ways to create longevity and will address some fears you may have as you wrap up this book. If you need to review the book, do so in a way that makes sense for you and your life. We will address some things that may make it difficult to create longevity and we will create some of the fears that you may have moving forward.

Application for the Future

CHAPTER 23

A LETTER TO STUDENTS AND YOUNG PROFESSIONALS

Veterinary school (and Technician school) is hard for a number of reasons. Aside from the academic rigor, you are also learning a new task. You are not going to be perfect at this new task. However, you are held to high standards of care. You likely have imposter syndrome. This is normal and also very hard to manage. Please be kind to yourself during the early stages of your career. The best learning is achieved by doing, which means you will have to learn from what not to do as well as what to do. You entered this field for a reason. Unless it is for the money, in which case you will likely be disappointed, hold this reason tight. It is easy to lose it in the first few years of work.

As you read this book, you may become discouraged. You will read about the mental well-being struggles in the field. It can feel like you are doomed. You are not. The changes are happening with your generation of veterinarians. Building resilience now is what is needed as you grow up in the field. Yes, this is a hard job. It has a lot of emotions tied to it, but it is worth it when you know how to manage them as they arise.

Building resilience is much harder than living in resilience. I know that this can seem weird in the moment, but please trust me. Your resilience skills may change as you grow in the field, but having a strong foundation will make you more likely to thrive when things get the hardest.

Enduring the hard and knowing it will get easier is the hardest part of getting through the first few years as a veterinarian. Find mentors and trusted people in the field to support you. They have been through it and come out of the other side. Not only can they give you advice as you grow up, but they can also give you hope that it will get easier. It can be hard to find the courage to establish these relationships. More seasoned professionals may feel intimidating, but for some, giving to you is just as rewarding to them as it is to you. Find those people.

It is unlikely that people find their dream job as their first job. Entry-level positions often have some extra stressors for them. Please understand that this is a learning position. You will be a better professional later in your career after having this position. Having a goal for what you would like your next steps to be and knowing this is a step toward larger goals can get you through the hard work of a first job in the field.

I hope you can look back in 5 or 10 years from now and cherish this time. You are learning and growing in a way that will set you up for future success. You are building a foundation for your future. Give yourself a pat on the back. Giving yourself space to take pride in your accomplishments is important. It reminds us that we worked for what we are, and it was worth it.

Don't give up. You might find this is more than worth it. If you build your skills both mentally and professionally, and use this time for growth, you will relish in your future success.

CHOOSE YOUR OWN ADVENTURE

Many of the exercises discussed in this book can be applied in various situations, not just the chapter in which they are. A skill addressed in Chapter 5, connection, may also be used in communicating with a handler or managing anger. I placed the exercises in the book where you can use them most effectively, but they can be applied in various ways. For this reason, I encourage you to review the skills and decide what you would like to try first, given your current struggles.

It is important to remember that we can only control our thoughts to a certain extent. You may notice some of the skills are more thought-oriented, even though the primary focus is on nervous system responses. This is because our thoughts and our bodily reactions are constantly communicating. If you think about something sad, your body responds with sadness. If your body is responding with sadness, your thoughts will likely be sad as well. Because our body's main goal is to stay alive, it responds and sends thoughts that it thinks we need to live. While thoughts and nervous system skills are both important in building resilience, we often notice the thoughts we have way more than the body sensations. If we lean into the responses of the body and find safety there, our thoughts are likely to shift. These skills can reset your nervous system. The idea is to address workplace stress from the perspective of managing the body's reaction, so that the mind can agree. As I mentioned in the introduction, I provide a range of various ways in which you can manage your emotions effectively. I do not expect that every skill will be helpful for every person. Some experimentation is necessary to determine what works best for you as an individual. It is important to try skills more than once to ensure that you are using them in a way that they have the potential to be effective for you. If you notice avoiding a skill, you can decide if it's time to move on and go back to this skill at a different time, or if it's better to explore why you are avoiding the skill and learn steps to get to a place where you can try it. You get to decide.

It is hard to apply skills in day-to-day life. It feels like you do not have the time and energy to build the skills. Sometimes it feels hopeless. While applying skills and building resilience is hard, it is far less hard than living in misery. Make it a priority for a month or two, and you will notice that changes will be made. As you build a foundation for well-being resilience, it creates plywood that covers up the hole that you can dip into with workplace stress. The skills become easier, and work becomes more manageable. You just have to get through the hard to get to the easy.

WHAT DO I DO IF SOMETHING IN THIS BOOK HELPS IMPROVE MY LIFE?

The answer to this question seems simple. You keep doing it. However, that is often easier said than done. It is not uncommon to find some really wonderful life-changing skills, and when push comes to shove or the shit hits the fan (however you would like to say it), you will naturally go back to the default mode before. This is because the default mode works in some capacity and can take less energy. The downfall is that it often has consequences. I encourage you to find some way to check in on the skills that work to ensure you are still using them. A first step would be to make a list of what works. During really difficult times in our lives, we often forget everything that ever worked. It is important to put it in your handwriting so that you can remember that it was you who liked these skills and found them useful, not someone else giving you "shoulds." I even know people who have made videos of themselves talking about what works and how they do it, so they can remember that they liked it at one point in their lives.

The next step would be to find a way you can check in with yourself. This may look different for everyone. I personally like to have several ways because I know that one, if not many, will be forgotten during difficult times. The most effective way to check in on yourself is to recognize your body's natural warning signs. This could be when you become more irritable with people, when you have the thoughts "this sucks", or when you want to stay in bed for more than one well-deserved lazy day. Everyone has their individual warning signal. I call my warning sign, "powering up." It is when I put my head down, work quickly and frantically, and try to accomplish all the tasks at once. Pay attention to the behavior, thought, or body sensation that you have that says, "Hey you are not grounded, go back to the basics." I encourage you to find something that you can notice before it gets gigantic. For instance, notice the slight annoyance that is relatively benign, not just the full-on rage over something disproportionate to the reaction. If you happen to miss the small, only become aware when the big ones show their ugly head, that's fine too, it is progress if you notice it, no matter when you do, and next time you are likely to notice it sooner. Making a plan for the hard times, using the skills that work for you, builds your resilience even further.

I also have important moments throughout the year that I check in on my well-being. Many people do this during the New Year season so that it comes naturally. I also check in on myself during my birthday and a few other holidays that my family celebrates, which knocks me off my routine just enough to check in. I encourage you to find times of the year for yourself as well. Check in during difficult times, such as anniversaries of challenging events in your life, and the middle of the season you dislike the most. Also, check in on less challenging times like the first of the year, a change in fiscal year, or anything else that jogs your memory to check in.

Lastly, I check in on myself as I enter my office. This is the most important and the check that takes the least amount of time. It has become a habit to check in on how I feel as I open the office door and turn on the lights. Do I think an "ugh, I do not want to be here." Do I feel grounded with the tasks I have at hand today, or am I thinking of the 8million things on my to-do list, both personally and professionally? This check-in allows me to identify which skills will be most important to use that day. I encourage you to do the same. These check-ins keep our skills constant so that we are less likely to forget them when they are most needed. They also allow you to catch the difficult times before they get too big.

Your check-ins will likely look different from mine, so please be creative with how you would like them to appear. Also know they may be clumsy at first. You will likely forget or notice too late as you start the process. That is okay. Because there is natural positive reinforcement in going back to the basic skills that work for her, and noticing when you are out of your window, your body appreciates it, no matter when you notice you are out of sorts, and is more likely to recognize it earlier the next time. Thank goodness for natural rewards. As you find things that work, applying them regularly will make them become a habit.

WHAT DO I DO IF NOTHING WORKED IN THIS BOOK AND I STILL FEEL STUCK?

Please do not feel discouraged just because the skills in this book did not speak to you. There are several reasons why these skills may not be effective.

You may have had a hard time applying the skills to your day-to-day life. If you did not use them, please find a way to make them smaller and more manageable. Be creative in how you can apply them, and be curious about what got in the way of application. If you just don't feel like you have time, find the skills that take up the least amount of time to start. If you want to, but it feels intimidating, find some way to apply them anyway. Building resilience does not happen until you do the work.

For some people, there is a fear of getting better or being calm. This is not a logical fear; it is a body reaction to messaging from somewhere in your life that communicates that getting calm or getting better will be dangerous. Sometimes, people worry that the other shoe will drop. At other times, there is something they will miss out on if they do not experience the uncomfortable feeling. It sounds weird, but our body reactions often are. When things have been a struggle for so long that it feels scary when skills finally work. Our body feels like it is dangerous to feel better. It fears you might miss something, and the unknown is always scary, even if it is for the best. If this is you, I encourage you to find a therapist who is a good fit. There are many different types of therapy, so if you find someone who is not understanding of the barrier, try out someone else. These types of barriers are extremely difficult, if not impossible, to work through on your own.

For some people, there is something deeper, and the skills only scratch the surface of a deep pain. In these cases, I also encourage you to find a therapist, but you may be looking for a different type of therapist. A trauma therapist who specializes in a modality that specifically treats your life may be the best fit for you. It can be amazing what processing trauma can open up for you. I like Eye Movement Desensitization and Reprocessing (EMDR), but several very effective trauma treatments can be life-changing for those who are struggling with deep pain from their past.

Sometimes the skills don't work because we just don't vibe. When it comes to work on well-being, there will be people you can relate to, and there will be people you just don't. Not everyone likes my teaching style or the type of skills I provide. That's okay. Explore some other well-being resources and see what might be more helpful for you. There is something for everyone; you just need to find out where you connect.

For some people, the number of skills was just too much. I give a huge number of various kinds of skills in this book. I recognize that this can be overwhelming for some, especially those who want to try everything all at once. I encourage you to try smaller ones if you are feeling overwhelmed by the skills. Pick 1–5 and apply them to the best of your ability. I know this can be counterintuitive, given that you likely want to find the skills that work yesterday if you are already struggling with burnout, but I can assure you that slow really is fast when we are speaking about well-being. Patients and moving slowly will allow for faster movements toward change. If you are uncomfortable with the slow pace of the skills, you are likely uncomfortable with any slow pace in life. You can start with struggles with slow and use skills there, if this is true for you.

Your work environment may be a barrier to wellness. However, I encourage you to wait to quit until you can make an effort to find grounding in the field. Some people need to make changes to feel better. The values of the clinic you are working for or the job you are doing are not coordinating with your own personal boundaries, which can interfere with any of the skills you could apply. If your resentment for your current position is very strong, it can be hard to work through this struggle. It is okay for a job not to be a good fit. This does not mean you are doing something wrong, nor does it mean they are either. In many ways, our jobs are similar to relationships. Sometimes we are in a relationship that just isn't a good fit. It gets in the way of our personal growth, and it is no one's fault. You are allowed to leave and find a different position if this is a barrier to your well-being.

No matter what the reason is for the book not applying to you, do not lose hope. I have met many people in my career who feel like change is hopeless. They feel stuck in the life they are living because therapy hasn't worked for them in the past. They find hope, change, and resilience in a new and different kind of therapy. There are so many therapist styles out there; please don't give up.

HOW DO I KEEP A BAD DAY FROM BECOMING WORK-RELATED STRESS?

We all have a bad day. Sometimes, a lot of bad things happen in one day. Sometimes, our system does not handle the stress and the stories the same way it may on another day. This can occur for a variety of reasons. Maybe you are more tired, or your hormones are wacky, or you were reminded of something else at some point in the day and didn't realize the situations were overlapping. Trying to figure out why the bad day is bad does a little. It helps you learn how to take care of yourself so that you can be more aware the next time, but the helpfulness of the why stops there. Sometimes we can crawl down the "why rabbit hole" so deep that it actually becomes a distraction from coping.

If you notice that your nervous system is activated and you are having a difficult time coming down from your day, don't go for the bottle, or drown yourself in clinic notes. Instead, take a moment before you leave the clinic. Take note of the fact that you feel unwell, and maybe it is understandable, maybe you aren't quite sure why. If you are feeling shut down, have a warm liquid. If you are feeling activated, do a couple of jumping jacks or drink a cold glass of water. Take a moment to check in with what your body needs in this moment. The skill you use may be magical and work wonders, or they may just turn it down a notch, and that's okay. When you begin your commute, start with the first half of your commute and ask yourself a few questions that can fill your brain with more than just thoughts about the crummy. What did I learn today? What went well today? Who did I make a difference for today? If none of these practical questions work, ask some more logical questions: how many B's can I find on license plates? Can I make a rainbow with the colors of the cars I see? Can I make the alphabet with random letters that I see? The point is to fill your brain with a different kind of thought. Then spend the second half of your commute deciding what you would like your home life to be like today. How do you want to act when you walk through the door? There is no correct answer here. There are some that are technically better coping mechanisms. My hope is that using the previous skills will enable you to adopt more effective coping mechanisms naturally. You may decide to relax when you get home after a hard day. Make your easy meal, watch trash television, and go to bed, telling everyone you are not available today. You may decide to leave work alone, push it to the side, and be the best person you can be when you get home, as if the day did not impact you. If you decide on this one, make sure you check on your hard day before you go to sleep or the next morning. You may decide something in between. You're going to be available to your family when you get home, make an easy meal, and go to bed early. Again, there is no correct answer; planning for how you want to be allows time to prepare for home life.

When you have a bad day, it is okay to chalk it up to a bad day. You can be the most effective person ever and use tons of skills, and there will be days when they work a little less. There will be days you forget to manage your stress, and it will catch up to you when the door locks. There will be days when there are more tough cases than you expected, people are bigger jerks than usual, or your colleagues around you are downright bitches. Let a bad day be a bad day; it doesn't have to mean anything at all. If you have two bad days in a row, it may be a rough couple of days. Don't forget to go back to what works for you, but there is no reason to be concerned about a few bad days. If your bad mood continues to linger for weeks, it might be time to pay attention. You may want to start asking yourself if you are struggling with your job, or certain cases, or compassion. If your bad mood continues to linger for more than two weeks, it's time to really double down on skills because you may be in the danger zone. Being in the danger zone of burnout is not a bad thing; it is just something to listen to. You may need to practice a few additional skills or consider reaching out to a mentor or therapist. You can get out of it much easier if you catch it earlier. The job is not unsafe yet; your system is just deciding if it is safe or not.

WHAT SHOULD I DO IF LIFE BECOMES DIFFICULT WHILE I AM WORKING THROUGH THIS BOOK?

As you work through this book, you will likely have some life stressors come up because it is impossible to pause life just to figure out burnout or work stressors. I wish we could pause life and pick it back up when everything is in order and ready to go, but that is not realistic. If/when life becomes challenging while you are exploring this book, I encourage you to use the same skills. To some, this may be a frustrating answer, but I am confident that if you use these skills to whatever capacity you are able, they will benefit you. Sometimes, when life gets hard, it feels like you have less capacity to apply skills. If you can give it 10%, you will benefit from them about 10% which in turn is doing 10% better than you were without the skills. This 10% begins to give room for 12%, and eventually, you may feel like you have the capacity to manage whatever life is throwing at you, even if it is terribly painful and downright sucks.

Being realistic with yourself is key here. If you try to give 100% and end up giving 10%, you are left not only with the difficult emotions that life throws at you in the moment, but also with shame that you are incapable of giving more than 10%. There is just one more emotion, jumbled up in the mess. If you check in with yourself and realize you cap out at 7%, you do the skill with the reality that you will probably be doing it at 7%. If you accidentally give it 10%, you now feel accomplished, knowing that you did more than you thought was possible. You receive positive reinforcement for the skill you're working on, and bam, you have built a new neuropathway in the brain. A habit is beginning to develop.

I know this takes patience, and patience downright sucks when things are hard. It is likely that at some point, while trying out the skills in the book, you will accidentally try to give it 100% and realize only after the fact that you were being unrealistic with yourself. Instead of being hard on yourself for being hard on yourself (hello, shame monster), just notice it as information. Okay, so I wanted it to work magically; it worked in a helpful way, but not as big as I had hoped. That could be worth it, and it could grow. Let's keep going and try for a little longer.

Now, if it is working at 0%, this does not mean that you are giving it 0% effort or that you are 0% good at this stuff. It simply means that this particular skill does not work for you. This provides you with valuable information that allows you to set that skill aside for now or forever (depending on your current feelings) and move on to the next skill in the book.

I can't stop life while you work through burnout or add resilience skills to your arsenal. Life is still happening. Stress will still come up. Sometimes, it involves really big stress and extreme transitions. I encourage you to keep on trucking through. Use the amount of energy you can to implement new ways of being. Give yourself grace within the hard without giving up. I have seen it pay off for people, and I believe it will pay off for you, too.

FOOD FOR THOUGHT JOURNALING:

1. How am I doing with the skills and concepts discussed in this book?

2. What is my plan moving forward now that I have digested the information in the book?

3. How am I feeling right now? How do I want to feel next week (realistically)? How do I hope to feel next month (realistically)?

LEARNING FROM THE PROCESS

As you go about this process, you likely found some techniques to get you out of burnout or build resilience. You likely also found some skills that did not work. If you gave this book time and really explored its possibilities, it is likely that some kind of intense struggle arose at some point while exploring this book. Some difficult cases came into the clinic, the ugly side of the dynamic and culture of veterinary medicine came to the forefront, or you no longer feel like your job is a good fit. It is important to learn from times when you struggle. Ask yourself what you saw in yourself, how you acted, and how others treated you. This becomes great information for the future to ensure that you pull out your note card and use the skills you are forgetting to use. You will have more stressful days, you will become irritable with people at some point, you will mess up, but use it as information.

Each time a skill works, you build a pathway in your brain that makes you want to do it more. It is positive reinforcement. Eventually, your body and your brain agree that being effective actually works better than whatever your default mode has been up until this point. You learn from the process of things working. You can't fight this process. You got into the habits you are in now because something worked (even if it has long-term consequences). Now we are creating new habits that work (with the hope of few if any consequences.)

You may do some of these skills without even thinking about it. Some of them likely come naturally. However, they are not coming to the forefront at the times you need them most. Intentionally applying skills where they are not already being used allows you the space to apply the stuff you are already doing to times when it may also be effective to use them. Some of these skills seem simple, and it can be very frustrating when they are harder than you think they should be. No matter how simple or complex a skill is, the application is the hard part. You are fighting the default mode that your body has established based on the experiences it has had up until this point. At some point, your default mode worked, and you can appreciate it for that, but short-term gain often has long-term consequences. Be patient with yourself. Change is easier said than done.

LEARNING FROM THE NOT-SO-GOOD

Past career stress can become a current trigger. It's annoying but true. If you become burnt-out, start feeling compassion fatigue, or develop symptoms of vicarious or secondary trauma, it is not comfortable. It is stressful just to have the symptoms. People often feel helpless, stuck, and, dare I say, broken in this moment. The feelings are not true, but they feel like it. Because this is a stressful time in your life, it can become a stressor that triggers future emotions.

It is common for people to come to me terrified that they are going to get symptoms of vicarious trauma due to a difficult case, when in fact they are not. They felt vicarious trauma before and fear that they will experience it again. When moments are difficult in life, people start to fear that burnout is on its way, especially if they have survived burnout in the past. This is a difficult concept because you absolutely want to catch symptoms before they get gigantic; this is vigilant. However, being hypervigilant (a little too much caution) leaves little space just to be well. Living life well is just as important as growing and striving to be better. We need the balance between the two.

When striving to grow and build yourself, it is important to know that you can have too much of a good thing. I have met people who I would define as being addicted to self-help and growth. It looks really good on paper. They are constantly growing and striving to be better. Reading the next self-help book and listening to the next podcast. However, self-help can become an avoidance of itself when the concepts are not applied. You can spend so much time learning how to be better, but you avoid the place you are in now. Sometimes, the place you are in now is painful and needs a different kind of working through. Sometimes it is not painful at all. It is neutral or good, but there is fear that it is not good enough, or if you acknowledge the good, it will go away. Sometimes the self-help addiction is because it is more enjoyable to listen to the best way you could live, than working hard and applying skills to change the way you are living.

I encourage you to spend some time exploring the balance between being just okay or good and striving to be better. Find some time for both. Maybe you give yourself a break from all the growing stuff and say, for the next month, I am just going to be and see how it goes. At the end of the month, take a moment to check in on yourself. "How am I doing?" "No, how am I really doing?" I say it twice because we are so used to saying "fine" or "good" when someone asks how we are doing that it is a habit to say it to ourselves. If we ask twice, we actually answer. Sometimes we need to ask three or four times to get a truthful answer from ourselves. If you are still doing pretty well: you are using skills naturally, feeling resilient, and overall feeling like things are going the way you would hope for them to go, great, take another month. If you check in and find that there is some sticky, yucky emotional stuff that you have not worked through. Something is making life pretty hard right now. Great, that is good information to go back to the working through stuff. The good news is you gave yourself a month to see if it is really there. Watch out for shame; it can arise in this situation. Remember, it is not a bad thing to be struggling; it is just information about what you need to work through (I wish I could convince everyone to believe this to their core, but that shame even comes up for me sometimes).

Please know that this does not mean you should plug your ears and pretend not to listen if you come across a really cool quote, podcast, or any other message that resonates with you throughout your life. You are still allowed to grow during your growth break. Please remember to hold the intention of the law (not obsessing over growth to the point where you cannot just live) and not the letter of the law (no learning and growing ever).

Timing your growth break effectively is very important. It can be helpful to talk to a therapist, coach, or trusted person to see if it is a good time for your growth break. If you are in a mental health crisis, please do not choose that time to take a break from growth. If you are having suicidal thoughts, struggling to function, or having difficulty carrying out important daily tasks, please find support. If you are in the throes of burnout and struggling to find purpose in your life, it is also not a great time to take a growth break. This break is intended for a time in your life when you feel like you have mostly established a routine that fosters resilience.

FOOD FOR THOUGHT JOURNALING:

1. Pulse check: How am I doing right now with my well-being? How am I really doing?

2. Where am I seeing myself thriving?

3. Where do I need to exercise caution and awareness?

FINDING WORK–LIFE BALANCE AS YOU GROW

While you are working, there is still home life, and while you are living life, work is still happening, isn't that annoying? People often talk about the necessity for a work–life balance. I wish things were always balanced, but unfortunately, this is not very realistic. Sometimes we need to focus more on work than on home, and sometimes we need to worry more about home than we do about work. It makes it super annoying to work through this struggle because, with the flexibility, also comes a lack of defined answers to resolve the issue. It is essential to have a way to manage your stressors so that you can excel in both your job and personal life.

EXERCISE 23.1 Getting stuff done

1. Make a list of activities that you must complete on a day-to-day basis for you to be effective at work. This would not be related to each client, as that could differ each day. These could be things like progress notes, checking in during commute, or checking email.

2. Create a list of tasks you must complete at home to be effective. What are your responsibilities, spoken and unspoken?

3. Looking at both lists, is it realistic that you can accomplish most of both lists as needed? If it is not possible to complete these tasks, you are setting yourself up to fail. Ask someone to pick up some slack in some of your responsibilities. If it is doable but overwhelming, move to the next step.

4. Create a time schedule to accomplish these tasks. Lay out a visual of what makes this possible. Ensure that skills for well-being are incorporated into the task list. They are just as important as all the other things.

5. Practice trying to accomplish each task mindfully. This means only focusing on that task. If that is difficult for you, you can fill

your brain with thoughts about that task. Consider labeling your senses. If you are washing the dishes, you are thinking about what the soap smells like, what it feels like to whip the dishes down (physically, not emotionally), and what your next step is, even if you have done it so many times you could do it in your sleep. Your brain can only think one thing at a time, so fill it with thoughts about the task.

6. See how your overwhelm feels. If you are still feeling overwhelmed, go back up to step three and assess if you are being realistic with yourself. Is there anything that you can do to reduce your stress? Is there anyone you can ask for help? If the answer is no, rewrite your schedule. Find a way to make it realistic, even if it is uncomfortable, and ensure you incorporate some of these skills into the mix so that you know you can manage it all.

EXERCISE 23.2   Checking in on your balance

Without a defined answer about how balanced you are, how do you know if you are spending too much time at home or too much time at work? It is so easy to feel guilty when you need to spend more time at work, and guilty again when you need to spend more time at work. Remember that guilt will not kill you. You are allowed to feel guilty. This exercise can allow you to survive guilty because you can make your decision based on logic.

1. Review the values you developed. It is essential for you to utilize your values in this exercise.

2. Check in with who needs you most right now. (I encourage you to journal about this because you might go back and forth with everyone needing you.)

3. How does your work feel when you spend time with your family? How does your family feel when you spend time at work? Sometimes our perceptions of needing to be everywhere at once are distorted, and people are more understanding than we assume.

4. Use the information from 1 to 3 and check to see if your guilt is justified. Are you indeed spending too much time at work and leaving your friends hanging? Are you ditching long hours at work to go home, while other people pick up your slack?

5. If you feel that your guilt is justified after going through these steps and fact-checking, make the necessary repairs and implement the required changes.

6. If your guilt is not justified, remind yourself that it is not justified, and you will survive it and continue to do what makes sense anyway. The more you tolerate guilt, the less intense it becomes.

HIT THE GROUND RUNNING

Now is the time to hit the ground running. You read the book. Hopefully, you worked on some skills along the way. You may have developed a plan for your next steps in skills. Regardless of your stage, ensure you follow through and remain consistent. Resilience and repair are not one-time lessons. It is something you need to do time and time again. You need to mess up, start over, and do it again over and over again. You can do this, and it is worth it, but I am not going to lie: It is stinkin' hard. Thank you for taking the time for yourself. That is the first and hardest step. You have realized you need the skills and started to learn about them. I encourage you to take the next step now. Thrive!

FOOD FOR THOUGHT JOURNALING:

1. What barriers will get in the way of success? How can I plan for them?

2. How do I feel about applying these concepts to day-to-day life? Is there any caution for change?

3. Where do I see myself in 5 weeks? 5 months? 5 years?

4. What can I do to remind myself about well-being tasks when they get forgotten in the day-to-day grind?

5. What are the most valuable things I learned from this book? How can I keep the value of these concepts?

6. What are the things that I did not connect with as well? Do I need to revisit these concepts as I grow, or leave them?

7. What is my plan for hard days?

8. What is my plan for hard months?

9. What gives me the most energy in my professional life? How can I focus on the things that give me energy?

10. What was I already doing that created positive well-being before I even picked up this book? How can I be consistent with those things?

Skills List

Chapter 17

Chapter 18

Chapter 19

Chapter 20

Chapter 21

Chapter 22

Chapter 23

Index